# Chasing Polio in Pakistan

# Chasing Polio in Pakistan

*Why the World's Largest*
*Public Health Initiative*
*May Fail*

SVEA CLOSSER

Vanderbilt University Press   NASHVILLE

This book is the recipient of the
Norman L. and Roselea J. Goldberg Prize
from Vanderbilt University Press for the
best project in the area of medicine.

This book is printed on acid-free paper.


Library of Congress Cataloging-in-Publication Data

Closser, Svea, 1978–
Chasing polio in Pakistan : why the world's largest public health
initiative may fail / Svea Closser.
p. ; cm.
Includes bibliographical references and index.
ISBN 978-0-8265-1708-1 (cloth : alk. paper)
ISBN 978-0-8265-1709-8 (pbk : alk. paper)
1. Poliomyelitis—Pakistan. 2. World Health Organization.
Global Polio Eradication Initiative. I. Title.
[DNLM: 1. World Health Organization. Global Polio Eradication
Initiative. 2. Poliomyelitis—prevention & control—Pakistan.
3. Health Policy—Pakistan. 4. International Agencies—organization
& administration—Pakistan. 5. Mass Immunization—organization
& administration—Pakistan. 6. Organizational Culture—Pakistan.
7. Poliovirus Vaccines—Pakistan. WC 556 C645c 2010]
RA644.P9C66 2010
362.196'835—dc22
2009041490

*For my parents,*
*with thanks and love*

# Contents

# List of Illustrations

**Figures**

**Photographs**

# Acknowledgments

I AM DEEPLY GRATEFUL for the extraordinary openness of people working at all levels of the Polio Eradication Initiative. The World Health Organization staff in Islamabad was particularly welcoming, and my work benefited enormously from the help and support of everyone there, particularly Dr. Obaid ul Islam, Dr. Nima Abid, and Dr. Javed Iqbal. I offer heartfelt thanks to these people for allowing me to work inside polio eradication, and for giving me the freedom to draw my own conclusions about what I saw. Many people in the Islamabad office taught and mentored me, but the analysis I present in this book is my own, and they bear no responsibility for the observations I present or the conclusions I draw here.

This work would not have been possible without the cooperation of the government of Pakistan. I am grateful for their permission to participate in polio eradication activities both in Islamabad and in three districts in Pakistan. In each of these districts, I was assisted by many people, but the exceptional support of the vaccinators Muhammad Kamran, Faisal Nadeem, and Sajjad Haider in arranging interviews deserves special mention.

Beyond Pakistan, officials at the World Health Organization in Geneva and the Centers for Disease Control and Prevention in Atlanta got me past their security checkpoints and answered my pointed questions with candor and thoughtfulness. Many anthropologists had assured me that these officials, who had nothing to gain by my knowing their business, would never grant interviews. Contrary to this dim anthropological view of the secretive development official, nearly everyone I spoke to responded to my intrusive and sometimes obtuse questioning with honesty and humor. For this I am grateful.

If the analysis I present here is critical of the Polio Eradication Initiative—and in many ways it is—it is because the openness and honesty I encountered deserves an open, honest response. The critiques I present here are given in the spirit of a colleague who believes in what these global health workers at all levels are aiming to accomplish, and who hopes that her thoughts on the subject may make their work a bit more productive in the future. I have taken advantage of my position as someone entirely outside the system to say things that people who work for global health agencies may not have the freedom to. In doing so, my aim is not to create problems for those who were so honest and open with me, but to assist them in their work by bringing some problems to light and suggesting possible ways forward. I deeply hope that proves to be the case.

In Pakistan, I benefited enormously from the help of a supportive extended family. Abdul Rehman, Khatoon Bibi, and Shamshad took care of my son better than I could have, cooked my meals, washed and ironed my clothes, walked with me to the bazaar at night when I decided I needed ice cream, and made sure I was entirely free to work in a way I am certain I never will be again. And they made it clear they did it out of love.

Nizakat and Farzhana too, along with their children, Hadia, Wishal, and Ali, overwhelmed me with support and love. Their apartment was in truth not large enough for the five of them, yet they embraced my frequent and lengthy stays. In the company of the beautiful, deeply moral, and wickedly funny Fari, I was always entirely at home. Fari, you've helped me more than you know, and if I could transport you to a house with a yard next door to me always, I would.

My research assistant, Tanveer Khan, was an invaluable help. His influence extends throughout this book. He, his wife, Rosina, and their three children welcomed me into their lives. So did Rabina Bibi, Samina Bibi, and Shabina Mumtaz. Shakeel ur Rehman also provided useful assistance.

It was not only in Pakistan that I was on the receiving end of extraordinary hospitality. In Geneva, Jamie Guth, Paul Bilgen, and Brendan Bilgen opened their lovely home to Kaif and me, and Paul spent many hours helping us discover Geneva. My time there was very special.

Part of what made my stay in Geneva so lovely was that I spent it with my mother, Sally Closser, who traveled around the world on short notice to watch my son so that I could get my work done. The physical and moral support that she and my father, Bruce Closser, provided was invaluable. Mom and Dad, thank you.

At Emory, a number of people helped me in my thinking and writing. Peter Brown constantly showed me ways I could improve my work while giving me the space to write what I wanted to. He is a truly exceptional mentor, and I am very fortunate to work with him. Joyce Flueckiger, Bruce Knauft, and Ron Barrett were excellent sources of constructive criticism and moral support. Prior to my research, Emory's Center for Health, Culture, and Society and Institute for Comparative and International Studies provided me with opportunities for making my thinking deeply interdisciplinary.

This book benefited greatly from the close reading and perspicacious comments of a number of sharp, funny, fabulous women. Tricia Fogarty and Elizabeth Milewicz read and made detailed comments on nearly the entire book, fixing problems both small and seemingly intractable. Seeing their faces pop up on Skype was often the highlight of my week. Erin Finley courageously took on the task of revising the final manuscript, providing clarity, motivation, and general genius. Anyone attempting to finish a book without an Erin is at a huge disadvantage. Hannah Burnett was a great sounding board, proofreader, and queen of graphical innovation: most of the charts and timelines in this book are thanks to her. Anne Barakat, Karen Bartlett, Jennifer Goetz, Maria Graham, Andrea Ward, and Amanda Young were somehow convinced that reading my page proofs would be a really fun activity on a night out.

A number of other readers too provided suggestions and insight that improved the book. The students in Peter Brown's seminar on global health at Emory University wrote me charming and useful letters about the draft they read. Judith Justice and William Muraskin provided thoughtful, doable suggestions that made the book clearer and more comprehensive. Michael Ames at Vanderbilt University Press was a supportive editor. Julie Solomon, Sarah Willen, Emily Proctor, Thurka Sangaramoorthy, Jennifer Kuzara, and Matthew Ryan listened to me whine and then gave useful advice.

Grants from the Wenner-Gren Foundation for Anthropological Research and the National Science Foundation funded this research. Emory University supported me generously and provided me with funds for a pilot study. Middlebury College provided money for additional exploration. And though perhaps I should be ashamed to admit it, PBS Kids helped me find time to write this book.

My son, Kaif, was an incredible travel companion. He approached every new experience, food, language, and method of transport with enthusiasm. As a toddler, he should have had every right to insist on routine, but in the face of endless travel and change he was flexible, open, and a complete joy. Kaif, I owe you. And given that in the course of this research you sat on my lap on sixteen long international flights, I'm glad you like airplanes so much.

# Chasing Polio in Pakistan

# CHAPTER 1

# Introduction

It's so frustrating! We know [what] is going to happen
and can do nothing to stop it!
—World Health Organization
(WHO) official, Islamabad

THE POLIO ERADICATION INITIATIVE, a twenty-year, six-billion-dollar project that has employed over two million people, is history's largest coordinated mobilization in the cause of public health. In 2001 alone, the Polio Eradication Initiative vaccinated about 575 million children against polio in ninety-four countries, most of them multiple times, and most by teams going door-to-door (World Health Organization 2002). Polio eradication may also prove to be one of public health's most spectacular failures.

The program is in trouble. After twenty years of work, the goal of eradicating polio has not been met. The program has made dramatic progress, reducing the number of new polio cases from hundreds of thousands per year in 1988 to around eight hundred in 2003. However, in the last few years the project has been unable to make significant headway in reducing the case count to zero; in fact, the number of new polio cases seen each year has increased.[1] In 2008, there were around 1,600 cases of polio in the world. Polio transmission stubbornly persists in four countries: Nigeria, India, Pakistan, and Afghanistan. With the two target dates set for eradicating polio already missed—2000, and then 2005—the possibility may be slipping away.

This book is an ethnography of the Polio Eradication Initiative as it played out in Pakistan in 2006 and 2007. It examines power relations and the politics of decision making in this major global health project, and describes the cultures of health systems from Geneva to the Pakistani Punjab. The central question this book asks is: Why does the effort to eradicate polio seem to be failing in Pakistan? I thought I might already know the answer to this question when I began my research. I thought that polio eradication officials would know little about local cultures, and I thought they would use local cultural beliefs as a scapegoat for failures of implementation. But as it happened, my preconceived ideas were wrong.

## Knowledge of Local Culture

It is a truism in medical anthropology that health projects often fail because they are based on insufficient knowledge of the cultures of the people they aim to assist. A common theme throughout the medical anthropology literature is the necessity of understanding local culture and beliefs in order to successfully implement health projects and effect behavior change (e.g., Hahn 1999; Paul 1955). Judith Justice's *Policies, Plans, and People* (1986) is justifiably a classic in the anthropology of global health and is the book that in large part inspired my own work. A central thesis of her work—one that holds true in many health projects I have observed in South Asia—is that the effectiveness of many health projects is limited by their failure to take local realities into account.

But the difficulties the Polio Eradication Initiative faces cannot be blamed on a lack of local knowledge. I was consistently impressed and humbled by how well Polio Eradication Initiative officials in Islamabad, and even Geneva, understood the complexities of local communities' attitudes toward polio immunization and the knotty dynamics of vaccination campaign implementation in district health systems in a variety of contexts across Pakistan. I had ingratiated myself into the project by offering to provide anthropological information that would expand planners' understanding of the people whose children they aimed to vaccinate, but I soon found I could tell them nothing that they did not already know.

Part of the reason people working on polio eradication had such deep knowledge is because of the structure of the project. Polio vaccination takes place in mass campaigns carried out over the course of about a week about eight times a year. During the campaigns, the World Health Organization offices in Islamabad emptied out save for a single employee charged with collecting the data arriving via phone, e-mail, and fax from various districts. World Health Organization and UNICEF employees fanned out across Pakistan, directly monitoring campaign activities in every district where cases of polio were still occurring.

A highly developed and sensitive surveillance system told planners exactly where polio cases were still occurring and thus where vaccination coverage was less than perfect, so they could focus their attention on places where quality was subpar. Because vaccination was not an ongoing activity but took place only on specified days a limited number of times per year, there was always someone present from Islamabad—and often from Geneva—to monitor activities in poor-performing districts. This prevented the phenomenon (well documented in the ethnographic literature) of short visits by high-level officials to easily accessible model sites where everything functions perfectly during the visits, leaving serious problems unobserved (Justice 1986; Mosse 2005). Since they had been visiting the same problematic districts over the course of nearly ten years of polio campaigns in Pakistan, officials based in Islamabad knew many areas of the country very well. They also had a thorough understanding of the reasons for low vaccination coverage in those areas.

High-level officials' depth of knowledge of local realities was also due to their extraordinary sophistication and dedication. For example, one high-level Pakistani WHO official who could cite anthropological literature on many areas of the country was, more importantly, humble, self-effacing, conversant in a number of languages, and prone to asking lots of the right questions. He and others in Islamabad had a wealth of local knowledge; the difficulties that the Polio Eradication Initiative faces cannot be blamed on ignorance on the part of policy makers and planners. People at all levels of the World Health Organization were open to and interested in an anthropologist providing cultural information which would benefit their project. But many of their own employees were de facto more experienced anthropologists than I, with my scant two years of experience in the country.[2]

## Blaming Culture

Anthropologists have also criticized global health practitioners for using the culture of local populations, when they pay attention to it at all, as a scapegoat for failed projects. What Paul Farmer calls the "conflation of structural violence and cultural difference" (Farmer 2005, 191) can deflect culpability for disease from those in power and place it instead on the poor. Public health planners (and others) may inappropriately attribute poor health outcomes to culture rather than to poverty. In *Stories in the Time of Cholera*, Charles Briggs and Clara Mantini-Briggs describe this process in a cholera outbreak in Venezuela. There, public health practitioners blamed the epidemic not on inadequate infrastructure or poor institutional response but on the putative cultural characteristics of the people who were dying in shocking numbers. The necessary corrective steps were never taken, and subsequently cholera again attacked the same populations. Briggs and Mantini-Briggs write that "assertions regarding cultural difference—the idea that poor people and individuals representing marginalized communities think and act differently and cannot embrace modern hygiene and medicine—increasingly shape institutional practices that permit or even multiply unnecessary and unconscionable deaths from disease" (Briggs and Mantini-Briggs 2003, xvii).

When I began my research, I thought I would find polio eradication officials blaming the failures of eradication in Pakistan on local culture. In interviews I conducted in Islamabad during a pilot study in 2005, I heard the "status of women" in Pakistan, as well as "corruption" in health systems, blamed for the difficulties the project was facing. But in spending a year immersed in polio eradication, I found that culture blaming was not a widespread practice. In retrospect, I suspect the people I spoke to early in my research searched for cultural factors to describe to me: they probably assumed that those were what I, as an anthropologist, would find interesting.

Cultural characteristics *were* often invoked as a reason for the difficulties in reaching certain populations. Take, for example, the following exchange between a supervisor and a vaccinator in a district in the Punjab:

> Vaccinator: There were two refusals in my area.
> Supervisor: Why did they refuse?
> Vaccinator: They're Pathan, sir.[3]

Here, that the people were Pathan—a minority group in the Punjab—was offered as sufficient explanation for their refusing vaccination.[4]

But this example is unusual. Overall, I was struck by the fact that whenever someone tried to blame failures of the campaign on the culture of the people in a given area, someone else almost always argued against them. For example, at one national meeting a foreign high-level official complained that, while in Iran and Egypt "people rush down to have their child vaccinated," in Pakistan "they go and hide the child from you." Several people at the meeting immediately argued against the implied ignorance and apathy of the Pakistani populace. They asserted that in Iran and Egypt, places characterized by decades of "world-class basic immunization," awareness of the benefits of vaccines would naturally be different.

Similarly, in a discussion in Islamabad about a remote district in the

North-Western Frontier Province (NWFP) that had recently experienced a polio outbreak, a senior official argued decisively against the cultural hypotheses being floated around. Two years ago, the area was a "model district," he argued. The culture hadn't changed, he insisted—the management had.

Most people at the highest levels of the Polio Eradication Initiative were dismissive of the idea that cultural barriers were insurmountable, placing the responsibility for reaching all populations squarely on the shoulders of polio eradication staff. A high-ranking WHO official in Islamabad told me he was skeptical of claims that polio could not be eradicated because of cultural factors. "It depends on our strategies, how we are approaching the people—there should be some ways to reach these people," he said. Another WHO employee in Islamabad said in a public presentation that putative cultural barriers in various areas of Pakistan were nothing more than an "excuse." Yet another reflected that "there is something *we* are not doing right in these populations." He caricatured the typical Polio Eradication Initiative supervisor getting out of a Land Cruiser wearing pants and sunglasses and talking into a cell phone, and the alienation that caused.

"It's true that the Muslim communities, particularly in Uttar Pradesh, have a higher incidence of polio than the surrounding Hindu communities," Olen Kew of the Centers for Disease Control said of the difficulties of reaching minority groups in India, "but it's not fair to point to any particular religious group as resistant to immunization because when those communities are approached appropriately, usually they welcome immunization" (Thigpen 2004). The blame for ongoing problems, then, lay with Polio Eradication Initiative employees for their failure to engage minorities "appropriately," not with the culture of marginalized communities.[5]

## Management Issues

Polio eradication leadership in Islamabad, for the most part, did not think that the difficulties the project faced stemmed primarily from the cultures of people living in areas with ongoing poliovirus transmission. Nor, as the quote that begins this chapter illustrates, did they feel that the failures of the program were due to a lack of understanding on their part about what was happening. On the contrary: they knew what the problems were, they knew what the solutions were. They blamed not the cultures of those receiving vaccinations, but the practices of district-level health leadership and other district-level government workers. They talked again and again about what they called "management issues." In districts with good "management," many opined, polio was gone; in those without it, children continued to be paralyzed.

If this assessment served to deflect responsibility from upper-level officials onto those with less power—and it probably did to some extent—it was nonetheless in large part accurate. As I mentioned earlier, polio eradication leadership in Islamabad, and even in Geneva, had an enviably precise and nuanced conception of what was happening on the ground. The leaders indeed did know what most of the problems were, and they were extremely good at predicting where polio cases would occur. But they were unable to translate this knowledge into a complete cessation of polio transmission. Many of these people were luminously intelligent and well informed, and all of them were extraordinarily hardworking. If *these* people couldn't eliminate polio from Pakistan, I found myself thinking, nobody could.

In this book, I explore and elucidate the "management issues" that make it so hard to stop polio transmission in Pakistan. These issues are in fact *resistance* on the part of district-level employees to the mandates of the Polio Eradication Initiative. As I will describe in detail, government workers resist in a number of ways, including foot-dragging, false compliance, and the use of networks of patron-clientism. This resistance—complex, diffuse, and without central organization—is a major reason that polio persists in Pakistan.

## Power inside the Project

This book explores the factors that made eliminating polio from Pakistan so incredibly difficult. At the center of the analysis are the complex interactions of donor, UN, and state power. Some anthropological explorations of development speak of "development discourse" or the "development apparatus" as if it were a coherent entity. But my work in the Polio Eradication Initiative suggests otherwise: not only is "development" not a unified whole, but this single development *project* is threatened by power struggles and contradictory agendas.

People who worked at all levels of the polio eradication hierarchy were acutely aware of these problems. What I write here will not surprise them. My contribution is twofold. First, I offer an analytic framework for what appeared to many in the project to be a diffuse set of intractable problems. The tools and the language that anthropology provides for dealing with issues of social organization and power relations are necessary for a clear exposition of what is happening inside the Polio Eradication Initiative. My aim here is to give health planners a language and a structure for understanding the internal dynamics of global health projects, to assist them in moving away from vague, imprecise terms like "corruption" and "management issues" toward conceptualizations of power and resistance that may concretely assist in better planning.

Second, I discuss publicly, and in writing, a set of issues previously limited to closed meetings and office gossip. The copious public documentation of the Polio Eradication Initiative does not address the internal power relations central to understanding its trajectory. Rather, in polio eradication's public façade, problems appear minimal or nonexistent. This book moves past the Polio Eradication Initiative's buffed exterior to describe its messy internal workings.

I do so not out of voyeuristic interest, and certainly not out of a desire to betray the trust of people who joked, a little uneasily, that I was "conducting surveillance" of them. I do so because internal power relationships are central to understanding why success was so elusive in polio eradication in Pakistan. If polio eradication fails, the analysis here will help explain the factors that stymied the best efforts of so many dedicated people. If it manages to succeed, the much more challenging eradication projects—of measles and malaria—that seem certain to follow on its heels will need to heed the lessons of polio eradication's difficulties if they are to have any chance of success. In this book, I introduce the concept of "political feasibility" as a way to think more clearly about the problems that eradication programs (and other global health initiatives) are likely to face. Critical analysis of international power relations and realistic assessment of how committed a given country's leadership is likely to be to a given health initiative are critical in avoiding the problems that currently plague the effort to eradicate polio. Anthropologists can contribute in important ways to such analysis.

## Anthropology and Global Health

Anthropologists working in global health largely fall into two general theoretical frameworks: anthropologists *in* global health and anthropologists *of* global health. I draw on both traditions in this book. Anthropologists *in* global health often work for development agencies and fulfill the role of culture broker, providing information on recipient populations to development planners in the hopes of making their interventions more effective (e.g., Brown 1983; Foster 1952; Hahn 1999; Paul 1955). Because they primarily work for global health agencies, anthropologists in global health may be wary of criticizing those agencies publicly. I did some work on vaccination coverage rates in nomadic populations moving through the Punjab for the Polio Eradication Initiative that fits securely into this tradition.

The anthropology *of* global health is anthropological study of the organizations that design, fund, and administer global health projects. The classic in this genre is Judith Justice's book that I mentioned earlier (Justice 1986). There has recently been an explosion of work in the anthropology of development agencies, and work on global health agencies—whose paradigms, structure, and sources of funding remain rather separate from those of development agencies more generally—is a growing field. But until very recently the literature on the internal workings of global health agencies consisted of three excellent articles (Nichter 1996; Pfeiffer 2004; Smith 2003); all three examine how local social relationships within health development projects affect the trajectories of these projects. The articles illuminate different aspects of global health projects—Nichter, for example, focuses on village-level primary health care staff, while Pfeiffer's analysis of the impact of the proliferation of nongovernmental organizations (NGOs) in Mozambique takes a national perspective. Each of these articles is a gem. However, given their short length, they are not able to describe in a comprehensive manner the complex interactions between different levels of a global health project, from donor to beneficiary.

The relationship between the two sorts of anthropologists described above—anthropologists *in* and *of* development—has often been strained. Anthropologists who work *in* development projects have been subject to some fairly severe criticism from colleagues in the academy who claim that they uncritically serve the interests of development projects, reinforcing global structures of power. Arturo Escobar, the most vocal critic in this vein, charged that anthropologists working for development projects "choose to remain blind to the historically constituted character of development as a cultural system" (Escobar 1991, 676). Escobar's condemnation of development anthropologists was tied to his conception of the nature of development as a whole. Elsewhere, Escobar argued that the discourse of development was totalizing and that, like Orientalist discourse, it "constituted a system for organizing the production of truth about the Third World . . . [which] made possible the exercise of power in novel ways" (Escobar 1992, 413; 1995).

Escobar's critique unfairly targets anthropologists who work for development agencies. Like the colonial framework of a century ago, the "development" framework is ubiquitous, and anthropologists—whether we work in development agencies or in the academy—cannot escape it (Edelman and Haugerud 2005; Ferguson 2005; Little and Painter 1995). Casting the debate in terms of "theoretical" versus "applied" anthropologists ignores both the contributions of theoretical anthropologists to systems of power and domination, and the possibility that applied work could make meaningful changes to those systems.

But Escobar has a point. Anthropology *in* global health, which tends to focus exclusively on the culture of recipient populations, can serve to blame the failures of health development projects on the poor or their "culture" rather than on global inequalities that structure their risk for disease and prevent them from accessing quality care. In doing so, it can reinforce the very disparities that lead to such shocking rates of disease among the world's poor (Briggs and Mantini-Briggs 2003; Farmer 1999; Nguyen and Peschard 2003; Singer et al. 1992). A productive way forward is to address how the cultures of development bureaucracies may be responsible for the difficulties many development projects encounter (Foster 1976, 1987).

The anthropology *of* global health is thus important. This book argues that the understudied internal workings of global health bureaucracies are key to understanding the failures of many global health projects. Global health philanthropy is currently in vogue: Bill Gates and Warren Buffett have thrown their fortunes behind it, and T-shirts funding AIDS treatment in Africa are available at the Gap. But there are complicated social processes that take place between, say, the purchase of an article of clothing in Michigan and the provision of antiretrovirals in Mozambique. If the promise of all this money is to be realized, the nature of these social interactions—and the ways in which they can stymie projects created with the best of intentions—must be understood. Anthropologists are ideally trained to carry out such analyses.

As an eradication program, the Polio Eradication Initiative is in some ways a special case. In important other ways—as a pioneering global health partnership, now the model for global health giving; as an internationally funded and administered project that works through government health systems; as a so-called vertical program (meaning it focuses exclusively on one disease)—it is similar to many of the largest projects currently under way in global health.[6] Understanding its pitfalls can, I believe, help us to plan better for the opportunities and challenges ahead.

In addition, this work makes contributions to the anthropology of development agencies more generally. There are a number of excellent ethnographies of development projects (Elyachar 2005; Ferguson 1994;

Hirschman 1967; Li 2007; Mosse 2005; Tendler 1975). These ethnographies have different foci, and none address directly and in ethnographic detail the power relationships between bilateral donors, UN organizations, and the national and district governments of poor countries. The work I was able to do is unique in its focus on global power relations *within* a development project. Such an analysis yields several important theoretical contributions. It allows a more nuanced conceptualization of "development," challenging the unstated assumption in some anthropological writing that "development" possesses a unified discourse. In addition, the multisited methodology and global focus of my project allow me to move past the general discussion of global "flows" that characterizes much writing on globalization and development to a specific ethnographic exploration of how global networks work (or don't work). This research is useful in understanding the success or failure of a given health development project but is also more broadly relevant, speaking to issues of sovereignty and power in the postcolonial era.

In doing so, it intersects with political anthropology. Aradhana Sharma and Akhil Gupta have formulated some of the questions driving current research in this field as "What would the state look like in a transnational frame where nation-states are not the only legitimate actors?" and "How does the transnational context impinge upon and redefine the ability of states to govern what is happening within their territorial borders?" (Sharma and Gupta 2006, 8, 24). There are many different answers to these questions, depending on the nation in question as well as the dimension of the "state" being considered. A number of recent articles have approached this problem using case studies of NGO and government development projects (Ferguson and Gupta 2002; Gupta and Sharma 2006; Sharma 2006). This book addresses these issues in a specific case. It illustrates how transnational power relations—such as those between a UN agency like the World Health Organization and a government like Pakistan—work in practice.

This book, then, is an ethnography of the Polio Eradication Initiative in Pakistan, approached in much the same way anthropologists have approached societies from the Trobriand Islanders to residents of the online community Second Life (Boellstorff 2008; Malinowski 1922). It is not an ethnography of Pakistani society in some broad sense. Very little of what most people in Pakistan do on a day-to-day basis has any effect at all on the trajectory of polio eradication, a project so focused that it takes only a few seconds of their time each month or so when immunization workers visit their homes. The problems the Polio Eradication Initiative faces are for the most part not to be found in the everyday lives or in the health beliefs of Pakistani parents—nearly all are perfectly happy to have their children immunized against polio, though it is not a priority for them. This book, then, includes a substantial amount of ethnographic detail on things that are extremely important in understanding why polio transmission continues in Pakistan—the thorny social dynamics of district-level health systems, the experiences of lady health workers, the complicated role of foreign consultants—and not a great deal on Pakistanis' lives more generally.

## Poverty, Inequality, and the Challenge of Eradication

Eradicating a disease—permanently stopping its transmission around the globe—is a difficult enterprise. It is difficult in large part because so much of the world lives in conditions of poverty that fan disease transmission. If the entire world had the same access to quality housing, basic sanitation, and routine immunization that citizens of the United States enjoy, polio would probably disappear on its own. But when so many people live in crowded and insect-permeable housing, without adequate systems for disposing of human waste or ensuring clean water, diseases like polio, measles, and malaria rage on.

That poverty promotes transmission of a number of diseases means that public health planners often must rely more heavily on biomedical interventions in poor countries than in wealthy ones, where many diseases common in poor countries are simply not public health issues. And these interventions may be less effective in poor areas: for example, to protect a child in India from polio may require three times the doses of vaccine required to protect a child in the United States (Grassly et al. 2006).

Close to one billion people on the planet live on less than one dollar a day (United Nations 2007). This poverty is tied to the wealth enjoyed by people in places like the United States. Global poverty is tied to the global economy, both its historical legacies and present configuration (Ferguson 2006; Wolf 1982). These global inequalities shape who is at risk for contracting disease as well as who gets effective treatment when they get sick (Farmer 1992, 1999).

A central argument of this book is that the same structures of inequality that keep disease transmission going in poor areas of the world *also* inhibit the effective creation and management of delivery systems that would aid in controlling these diseases. Power differentials between countries, including who is rich and who is poor, determine which global public health initiatives are taken on, how they are structured, and how they are viewed by both the populations on the receiving end and the ground-level workers implementing them. These dynamics, I will argue, are essential to understanding the trajectory of the Polio Eradication Initiative.

## Success and Failure

It is currently in vogue in the anthropology of development to eschew analysis of whether and how development projects meet, or fail to meet, their stated goals. Several prominent anthropologists have explicitly focused on the "side effects" or "tactics" of development projects rather than on their success or failure (Ferguson 1994; Li 2007, 231). Such scholarship has brought to light interesting and important effects of development projects and their rhetoric, and made it clear that development projects often serve to entrench existing structures of power. But the widespread nature of the current trend of neglecting to look seriously at success and failure is, to me, troubling.

The success of development projects in their stated goals is generally something to be desired. Poor people want to have more money, better food, and less disease—major goals of many development projects. If these projects fail, as they often do, it is important to understand the reasons for their failure.[7]

Many people writing in the field of critical medical anthropology have found a good balance: keeping global structures of inequality in view while not discounting the possibility that development interventions like vaccination campaigns can have real, positive effects even within those structures. Paul Farmer, for example, describes clearly the ways that structural inequalities structure health outcomes—and also argues persuasively that the major problem with biomedicine is that "there isn't enough of it to go around" (Farmer 1999, 14).

A critical eye for the ways that development projects may feed into larger structures of power need not preclude hope that these projects will succeed in making life a little better for poor people. Responsible, nuanced analysis can incorporate both. Insofar as anthropologists who have the freedom to work independently of the "development machine" can provide constructive criticism aimed at increasing the effectiveness of interventions, we have a responsibility to do so. And if a development project is making things worse for its putative beneficiaries, anthropologists have a serious responsibility not just to criticize but also to search for the way forward.

# The Pakistani Context

Pakistan is a large and diverse country with a population of around 170 million (and, more to the point for polio eradication planners, about 30 million children under five). It is bordered by Iran, Afghanistan, China, and India. Of these four countries, two—Afghanistan and India—harbor ongoing polio transmission. While Pakistan's sealed border with India keeps polio transmission from being shared between those two countries, the virus moves freely across Pakistan's porous border with Afghanistan.[8]

Pakistan is a nation of stunning contrasts. In Pakistan's Northern Areas, home to some of the world's tallest peaks, the climate is cold enough to support some of the world's largest glaciers, but in most of the country summer temperatures well over 40 degrees Celsius (104 degrees Fahrenheit) provide ideal habitat for the heat-loving poliovirus. Pakistan is home both to extremely remote, nomadic desert populations and to megacities like Karachi, with an estimated population of twelve million. The country's population is about 97 percent Muslim but otherwise diverse, with a wide variety of ethnic groups and languages. (Urdu, the national language, is almost no one's native tongue.)

The diversity—and, at times, disunity—of Pakistan's population is a product of the country's somewhat arbitrary creation when the British left India in 1947. The nation was originally conceptualized as a homeland for India's Muslims, and its boundaries were drawn to include most of India's Muslim-majority areas, in the process splitting culturally and linguistically coherent areas like the Punjab in two. When these borders were created, the horrific and unforeseen communal violence of Partition forced from their homes and across these new boundaries those who suddenly found themselves on the "wrong" side (Hindus in Pakistan, Muslims in India).[9] One Muslim-majority area, Kashmir, was assigned to India, and the ongoing dispute between Pakistan and India over whom the area rightfully belongs to has several times erupted into war.

Faced with the ongoing threat of conflict with India, several times larger than Pakistan in both area and population, the Pakistani government has placed a heavy emphasis on financing national defense, while sectors like education and health remain underfunded. In 2005, expenditure on health by the Pakistani government was just 1.5 percent of total government spending, one of the lowest percentages in the world (World Health Organization 2008c). These low public expenditures on health, coupled with high rates of poverty—the government estimates that over 30 percent of the population does not have enough money for adequate food (Government of Pakistan Planning Commission 2005)—help to explain Pakistan's unimpressive health indicators.[10] Nearly one in ten children dies before reaching the age of five; major killers include preventable, easily treatable diseases like respiratory infections and diarrhea (World Health Organization 2006e).

When I did my fieldwork in Pakistan for this project in 2006–2007, the country was in turmoil. General Pervez Musharraf, who seized power in a coup in 1999 (control of Pakistan's government has historically alternated between elected and army leaders), found himself facing threats to his legitimacy from several very different quarters. In early 2007, Musharraf attempted to remove the country's chief justice, Justice Iftikhar Muhammad Chaudhry, from his position, ostensibly because Chaudhry was corrupt (but actually, public opinion in my lower-middle-class neighborhood had it, because Chaudhry was in league with Musharraf's opposition and was sympathetic to constitutional challenges to the legitimacy of Musharraf's rule). Chaudhry refused to leave his post, and hundreds, perhaps thousands, of lawyers across the country staged street protests in his support. Rallies grew in size, violence, and incoherence, and fighting broke out on the streets of Karachi. About thirty people were killed, and the city was placed under curfew. (The polio vaccination campaigns planned in the city were postponed by several weeks.)

Almost simultaneously, Musharraf's government was engaged in a highly visible armed conflict with a very different type of opposition. In early July of 2007, government forces surrounded the Lal Masjid (Red Mosque), a large complex including a mosque and live-in madrassah on a tree-lined street in one of the wealthiest sectors of Islamabad. The leaders of the mosque and madrassah were militant Islamists, and over the past months the residents of the complex had become increasingly violent, kidnapping Chinese women that they claimed were prostitutes, setting fire to the inventories of several nearby video and book stores, and attacking a government office building. The standoff between government forces and the militants inside the complex went on for the better part of a week, during which time hundreds of students left the complex and—to the lurid fascination of all of us watching on television—one of the mosque's leaders was captured while attempting to escape wearing a woman's burqa. Ultimately, government troops bombed and stormed the complex, killing many of the people left inside.[11]

These very real challenges to Musharraf's position from such different quarters—the elite liberal intelligentsia represented by the lawyers (Dalrymple 2007) and the militant Islamists represented by the residents of the Lal Masjid—took place in the context of a country characterized by increasing disquiet, where suicide bombings killed civilians on a near-weekly basis. _Ḥālat kharāb hai_ [Things are bad], people said, shaking their heads, and scaled back their evening walks and trips to the crowded bazaars.[12] It seemed to nearly everyone I spoke to that Musharraf's days were numbered; many feared the country was slipping toward civil war. Musharraf had a great many things to worry about. It is safe to assert that the eradication of polio was not his top priority.

Musharraf's grip on the country progressively weakened, and in late 2007, after my fieldwork was over, he imposed emergency rule on the country. In August of 2008, he was forced to resign. Power transferred to Asif Ali Zardari, but this transfer is unlikely to have a huge effect on the trajectory of polio eradication in Pakistan. Like Musharraf, Zardari is verbally supportive of polio eradication efforts; like Musharraf, Zardari is in an extremely precarious political situation. The success or failure of polio eradication is not Zardari's chief concern.

In 2008, the Taliban took control of the Swat valley, in northern Pakistan, and (in contrast to earlier practice in many Taliban-controlled areas) decided not to allow polio vaccination there. While a setback to the program, this development is not the program's only problem, nor its most serious. The Swat valley is remote, sparsely populated, and cold—poor habitat for poliovirus. In 2008, poliovirus transmission intensified in all four provinces of the country, including fully accessible areas of the Punjab that had previously eliminated polio. The primary problem that the Polio Eradication Initiative in Pakistan currently faces, while exacerbated by the deteriorating security situation, is the same one it faced in 2007 when I did my research: an ongoing inability to carry out campaigns at the extremely high level of quality necessary to eliminate polio.

## Methodology and Position

The inherently global nature of a study of polio eradication necessitated an anthropological method somewhat different from that of classical ethnography, in which the researcher spends at least a year engaged in participant observation with a single community. Rather than produce a detailed ethnography of a single place, I aimed to develop a nuanced understanding of an entity, the Global Polio Eradication Initiative, that transcends a given locale. I was interested in the links between the local and the global, which required ethnographic research in a number of places, including communities on the receiving end of house-to-house immunization and surveillance, the local bureaucracies carrying out surveillance and immunization campaigns, and the offices of polio eradication officials in Islamabad, Geneva, and Atlanta. Such "multi-sited ethnography" has gained currency in anthropology as a way of describing issues tied up in the "world system" (Marcus 1995). In the course of my research, I "followed the project," analyzing the progression of Global Polio Eradication Initiative policy from Geneva to a city in the Punjab (Markowitz 2001).

In opting for multisited research, my goal was not to perform a comprehensive ethnography at each site. Rather, my aim was to gain a full understanding of the Global Polio Eradication Initiative, a complex project that exists across many locales. Multisited methodology, which requires spending a limited time at each site, does not necessarily lead to "thin" ethnography (that is, descriptions of events that lack a nuanced understanding of the context in which they take place). On the contrary, and as I had expected in designing this project, it was only through an understanding of what is happening in Atlanta, in Geneva, and in Pakistani cities that I could construct a rich, "thick" ethnography of events in Islamabad.

I spent one year doing fieldwork, more than ten months of which was in Pakistan. My central site was the Pakistani National Institutes of Health in Islamabad, home to the World Health Organization's Islamabad office and the government officials responsible for childhood immunization in the country. Both WHO and government employees were accustomed to foreign researchers visiting Pakistan to work on polio eradication for anywhere from a few weeks to a few years, and I was quickly assimilated into the role of "foreign consultant." I was given a desk in the National Surveillance Cell, invited to participate in planning meetings, and given free access to the Polio Eradication Initiative surveillance data and files, which included most of the reports and e-mails that had passed through Islamabad over the past five years. I spent a total of four to five months in Islamabad, conducting participant observation in meetings and daily office life. The environment in the office was collegial; I often ate lunch with the other people in the office, participated in office conversation and e-mail forwards, and assisted in the preparation of documents and presentations (where my being a native English speaker was useful). I attended the two weekly official meetings for polio eradication, as well as more formal events such as the Technical Advisory Group meeting, a two-day convening of epidemiologists, donors, and advisors from all over the world. Most of the meetings in Islamabad were in English; however, most office conversation was in Urdu, and my knowledge of Urdu was very helpful in understanding the dynamics of daily work in Islamabad.

In Islamabad, I conducted fifteen formal, semi-structured interviews, each lasting between thirty minutes and an hour, with WHO, UNICEF,

Rotary, and Pakistani government officials, as well as with representatives of major bilateral donors to polio eradication such as the U.S. Agency for International Development (USAID), the Canadian International Development Agency (CIDA), the Japan International Cooperation Agency (JICA), and the UK Department for International Development (DFID). These interviews, some of which I audio recorded, provided a useful complement to my observations in government offices. They also provided an interesting glimpse into the culture of bilateral aid agencies in Islamabad, one characterized by unmarked offices and metal detectors.

To better understand the process of policy implementation, I participated in four campaigns that aimed to immunize each child under five in Pakistan with oral polio vaccine. These campaigns, the backbone of the polio eradication strategy in Pakistan, are conducted approximately every two months and involve door-to-door vaccine delivery at every house in the country. The four campaigns were carried out in three Pakistani districts, ranging in size from around one thousand to around five thousand square kilometers with populations of between 600,000 and 3.3 million, according to the 1998 census.[13] My involvement in each campaign covered all stages, from planning to evaluation, and lasted about three weeks. Initially, I had expected to be a low-key observer of the campaigns. However, in every district I was rapidly pushed into the role of foreign monitor, a position with a great deal of power. I was whisked around in Land Cruisers, charged with presenting polio eradication "key messages" over tea to very powerful and highly placed government functionaries, and expected to present recommendations to the executive district officer of health. Government employees addressed me with honorifics that ranged from "madam" to "doctor sahib." Seasoned government officials became visibly nervous in my presence. The question of why a relatively inexperienced foreign student was given so much status is an important one that I address in further detail in the body of the book. I discuss other aspects of my participation in campaigns in Chapter 3, which is devoted to a detailed description of a campaign in a district I call by the pseudonym Kaifabad.

Kaifabad, a rapidly expanding megacity in the fertile plains of the Punjab, was the site of my most detailed investigation of the dynamics of project implementation. In total, I spent three to four months performing research there. In addition to participant observation in two campaigns in Kaifabad, I spoke with a variety of people involved in some way in polio eradication activities. I conducted and audio recorded individual semi-structured interviews of between five and forty minutes with more than twenty lady health workers in Kaifabad, and two focus groups of lady health workers that lasted about an hour each with a total of about forty participants.[14] While the lady health workers saw me as a representative of the Polio Eradication Initiative from Islamabad, most welcomed the opportunity to speak about their work with a woman whom they viewed as having the power to advocate on their behalf. These interviews, as well as much of my participant observation in Kaifabad, were carried out in Urdu.

In Kaifabad, I also conducted structured interviews with seventy-eight mothers of children under five, about half from nomadic communities and about half from lower-middle-class neighborhoods. These interviews were designed to produce information amenable to statistical analysis on how many children in these communities had been vaccinated. I also spoke to the mothers about their experiences with and attitudes toward the polio eradication effort. The interviews themselves, while fairly time-consuming to set up, in many cases lasted as little as five minutes; in rare cases, they could take half an hour. In general, I found that mothers did not have a great deal to say about the Polio Eradication Initiative; while it was part of everyone's life, it was not a major part of anyone's, and most mothers simply accepted polio vaccination without giving the matter much thought. Even my closest and most voluble friends did not have much to say on the topic.

At the time of my research, I was married to a Pakistani. In Islamabad, Kaifabad, and other areas of Pakistan, I stayed with his extended family, participating fully in local life in lower-middle-class neighborhoods. My family and friends knew that my research was on polio eradication, so this was often a topic of conversation. My brother-in-law, Tanveer, served as my research assistant, accompanying me in nearly all my work and providing me with friendship, respectability (women in Pakistan usually prefer not to travel alone), and an intelligent sounding board. He also transcribed recordings of Urdu-language interviews (transcribing interviews conducted in English was my responsibility). Tanveer's impish sense of humor and enthusiasm for his job enriched my research.

To better understand the culture and perspectives of the international health professionals who procure funding and create policy for the Polio Eradication Initiative, I conducted interviews, participant observation, and archival research at the WHO headquarters in Geneva and the headquarters of the U.S. Centers for Disease Control and Prevention (CDC) in Atlanta. In both places, my status was that of temporary visitor, someone who attended a few meetings and conducted interviews. People who worked in these offices spoke candidly with me and went out of their way to provide material—documents, data, and even in one case a poem—I would find interesting. In Geneva, officials whom I had met in Islamabad welcomed me and enabled me to make excellent use of a brief three weeks. Contacts at Emory University facilitated my research in Atlanta, conducted sporadically over the course of a year.

Throughout this book, I include myself in ethnographic descriptions of situations where I was present and provide the reader with personal information that shaped how others viewed me. In research driven by the personal interactions of participant observation and interviews, personality and identity matter: they affect the dynamics of interactions with others and thus the information a researcher can collect. As Lila Abu-Lughod writes: "We are always part of what we study and we always stand in definite relations to it" (Abu-Lughod 1990a, 27). These relationships and my position in them matter, and elucidating them is important.[15]

At times in the descriptions that follow, I may seem more critical of those lower in the polio eradication hierarchy than I am of those at higher levels. This is regrettable, but I can identify at least two reasons why it may be the case. The first is positional. In the course of participant observation, I was nearly always placed in a position of power. I am thus more acutely and personally aware of the pressures and limitations faced by people at higher levels of the Polio Eradication Initiative than by those at lower levels, which may color my perceptions. The second reason that this manuscript might be biased toward those in power is a problem of anthropological ethics. While the identity of a given vaccinator or other low-level worker can easily be disguised, given the vast numbers of such workers, camouflaging the identities of people at higher levels of the project is not so easy. While I use pseudonyms throughout this book, people inside the Polio Eradication Initiative will likely be able to identify many people I describe. While the events I write about are not secrets, I am wary of criticizing people in print—especially officials whose graciousness made my work possible and who might feel personally hurt by my judgments. Overall, my aim is not to be critical of the actions of individuals but to be critical in the sense of Merrill Singer's definition of critical medical anthropology, making a "theoretical and practical effort to understand and respond to issues and problems of health, illness, and treatment in terms of the *interaction* between the macrolevel of political economy, the national level of political and class structure, the institutional level of the health care system, the community level of popular and folk beliefs and actions, and the microlevel of illness experience, behavior, and meaning, human physiology, and environmental factors" (Singer 1998, 225). My aim in this book is to show how the actions of people at *all* levels of the Polio Eradication Initiative are connected to these larger systems.

Further description of my methods and position, and their implications, appears throughout the book whenever these issues become relevant. What I wish to emphasize here is that although my research took me to wildly divergent places (traveling straight from Kaifabad to Geneva and back gave me a case of economic and cultural whiplash), they were in fact deeply connected. Decisions made in Geneva affected the ability of lady health workers in Kaifabad to provide for their families; local politics, like those described in Kaifabad in Chapter 3, frustrated the ambitions of virologists in Atlanta. It was a privilege to have the opportunity to see the Global Polio Eradication Initiative in action in these diverse locations, and I strongly believe multisited research was the best way to understand the scope and contradictions of this immense and important project.

## Caveats and Limitations

Endemic polio exists today in four countries. This book is about only one of them. The discussion and conclusions of this book apply to Pakistan; I did not visit India, Afghanistan, or Nigeria, and in the case of Nigeria, at least, it appears that the challenges facing would-be polio eradicators are somewhat different.[16] Some of my conclusions, such as the effects of the culture of optimism, apply in all these countries; others, such as the nature of the patron-clientism in Pakistani districts, may or may not be transferable. It is likely that the resistance on the part of government health staff that I describe in Pakistan is a factor in other polio-endemic countries as well, but further research would be needed to confirm this hypothesis.

Pakistan is a large country. I could not visit all of it in the course of this research. While much of my research was carried out in areas where polio transmission had already been interrupted, it resurfaced in most of these areas in 2008, evidence that the difficulties in carrying out high-quality campaigns that I observed in 2007 and describe here had an effect. I also spent time, and worked on a campaign, in one of the country's worst-performing districts, tenuously protected from ongoing poliovirus transmission only by low population density and a cold climate. I had long conversations with many people who had spent a lot of time working on polio eradication in a variety of districts in Pakistan, and the problems they experienced, while exacerbated in some cases by serious security problems, did not differ greatly in nature from the ones I was familiar with.

The factors that I argue form the central explanations for the failure, thus far, of the elimination of polio from Pakistan—the ways that government employees may manipulate the system, the relationships between UN and government employees, and the power dynamics between the Pakistani government and UN agencies—are not unique to one area of the country.

## Outline of the Book

*Chasing Polio in Pakistan* explores the levels of the Polio Eradication Initiative, from vaccinators going door-to-door in rural Pakistan to planners preparing PowerPoints for donors in Geneva. In each place, I explore the culture, politics, and power relations that shape what people do. Ethnographic vignettes between the chapters illustrate how people at a variety of levels—from high-level officials in Geneva to mothers of young children—relate to the Polio Eradication Initiative. Polio is a tough disease to eradicate, but in theory, stopping transmission across the globe is feasible. The social relations I describe in this book explain why, thus far, this goal has remained just outside the realm of the possible.

Chapter 2 introduces eradication as a concept, and the history and structure of the Polio Eradication Initiative. It also introduces the Polio Eradication Initiative's culture of optimism, which I argue both sustains and hobbles the project.

Chapter 3 is an ethnographic description of my participation in an immunization campaign in a Punjabi district. Through a narrative of specific events, it brings up a number of issues that I explore more theoretically later: the role of the foreign consultant, patron-client relations in district health systems, and the techniques of resistance that district health staff use against supervision by UN agencies.

Chapter 4, which functions as a companion chapter to Chapter 3, explores these issues in theoretical terms. I look at the ways district-level health staff resist the mandates of the Polio Eradication Initiative, including falsification and lying; the use of patron-client relationships; and corruption. Staff resist for a variety of reasons, including dissatisfaction over low pay and their belief that polio eradication will never be achieved. In an attempt to cut through this resistance, UN employees use what I call everyday techniques of power, including propaganda, surveillance, and the construction of a parallel bureaucracy. Ultimately, however, these strategies of exerting power are insufficient to counter the effects of health staff's strategies of resistance, resulting in ongoing polio transmission in much of Pakistan.

Chapter 5 focuses on power relationships in the Pakistani capital, Islamabad. It explores the tension between the ideal that polio eradication is a Pakistani government project, and the reality that it is conceived, funded, and implemented by wealthy countries and UN agencies, with somewhat reluctant Pakistani government involvement. It explores the way that government employees at the *national* level resist UN mandates, and the techniques of power that the UN agencies use in attempts to get the Pakistani government to do what they want. While wealthy countries and UN agencies had sufficient power to get Pakistan to adopt the ambitious program of polio eradication, they are unable to make it the first priority in a country swamped with other problems.

Chapter 6 focuses on Geneva, dominated by the culture of global health, which vaunts collaboration and partnership as the key to solving the world's major public health problems. As a comparison case to the current quagmire in polio eradication, I describe the methods used in the successful Smallpox Eradication Program and argue that collaboration and partnership may not be enough to realize a goal as ambitious as eradication. I argue that the culture of optimism in Geneva, driven in part by a desire to keep donors giving, masks power relations and prevents honest and public discussion both about the problems facing the Polio Eradication Initiative and about what would be necessary to achieve eradication.

Chapter 7 presents my conclusions. I introduce the concept of political feasibility as an important determinant of the possibility of eradicating a given disease. I also suggest concrete steps to foresee and plan for problems like the ones polio eradication is facing. Assisting in such planning is a crucial way that anthropologists can contribute to global health.

The current era of vastly increased funding for improving the health of the world's poor is one of great potential. But to harness the power of all that money, we need delivery systems that work.

# Bus Number 11

Fatima is a lady health worker in Kaifabad. Because she lives
in an area of Pakistan where no new polio case has been seen
for several years, she works on three to five door-to-door polio
campaigns a year. In areas with ongoing transmission, lady
health workers work on six to eight polio campaigns a year; in
the winter, there may be a campaign every month. For each
campaign, Fatima must take about five days away from her
normal work and family life. Along with another worker, she
goes door-to-door in Kaifabad with oral polio vaccine, asking
if children under five are present and vaccinating them if they
are. At each house, she records on the door with chalk when
she visited, how many children under five live in the house, and
how many she has vaccinated. The areas she visits have been
carefully mapped out to ensure complete coverage of the city.
When Fatima comes to houses when the young children are not
home, perhaps at their grandmother's house or in the bazaar,
she records their names, ages, and the address and returns to the
house, often multiple times, until she finds and vaccinates them.
She does all of this, she notes, on "Bus Number 11," her own
two legs. As Fatima goes door-to-door, other teams of workers
vaccinate children at "transit points" like bus stations and busy
markets.

As a lady health worker, Fatima helps her neighbors with
a wide variety of health issues, from birth control information
to oral rehydration in cases of diarrhea to assistance with
tuberculosis treatment. Her salary for this work is Rs. 1,900
(around $30 a month). During the weeks of polio campaigns,
however, she focuses solely on polio and receives a supplement
of Rs. 600 (about $10) for five days of work.

Fatima is plump and talkative, with a sparkle in her eye. On
campaign days, she gets up at dawn for morning prayers and
then cooks breakfast for her husband and three children. She
irons her two older children's school uniforms, makes sure their

books are in their backpacks, and delivers her young daughter to the neighbor who will watch her for the day.

Depending on the area where she is working, Fatima may or may not have a proper lunch—if she knows people there, she may have lunch at a friend's house, but in areas where she is less familiar, she may not eat much. When Fatima gets home, she picks up her young daughter, goes over the day's homework with her older children, and cooks dinner for the family. She does the dishes. If the electricity is working in the evening, she irons her and her husband's clothing for the next day. She gets to bed late.

She describes a day of work to me:

> I start at eight in the morning and may not be done until four or five in the evening. We have to finish polio. We also have to mark the houses, and give the day's report to our supervisor. . . . When we're tired from the day's work we have to go back to the hospital to hand in our report. Then we have to go [to the hospital] early in the morning the next day to get vaccine, and then back to start working [vaccinating children]. After the day of work we go back again to hand in our reports. . . . It's really quite far. . . . It's all walking, walking. It's true that we do get lots of exercise—but that whole week I feel sick [*bukẖār nhīṇ utartā*]. Then, of course, we have to go back over those same areas to find the children who weren't there the first time. It's so tiring—I'm sure you know. And then everyone [the lady health workers] has to find someone to watch their children. . . . And the pay! You know about the pay.

## CHAPTER 2

# Polio Eradication in Policy

We will no longer have to live in a two-tiered world. And
I think that may be the single most important legacy of
polio eradication, the end of acceptance of what shouldn't
be acceptable.
  —Olen Kew, CDC

The only way to protect every child from polio is to
eradicate this crippling and potentially fatal disease
completely.
  —Bill Boyd, president, Rotary International

The eradication of a disease is the ultimate contribution
for sustainable health development.
  —Margaret Chan, director-general, WHO

ERADICATION, THE PERMANENT OBLITERATION of a disease, is a
powerful ideal.[1] Its supporters are impassioned and eloquent. It also has
a number of clear advantages as a public health strategy. Because the goal
is unambiguous and progress toward that goal is measurable—the case
count—monitoring performance and ensuring accountability are relatively
simple. If an eradication program succeeds, the disease in question ceases
to be a human problem, and in theory at least, the money and energy thus
saved can be used to address other health problems. Not least, as what Dr.
Margaret Chan calls the "ultimate" in public health, eradication attracts
supporters that more mundane control programs do not. But achieving
eradication is extraordinarily difficult.

## Eradication as a Strategy

Eradication is a very difficult endeavor, different from the usual public health goal of disease control. Control programs, the routine strategy in public health, aim to reduce incidence of disease to an "acceptable level." In contrast, eradication is the "permanent reduction to zero of the *worldwide* incidence of infection caused by a specific agent as a result of deliberate efforts; intervention measures are no longer needed" (Dowdle 1999, emphasis added).[2] When discussing eradication, health planners often also mention "elimination," a slightly different benchmark. Elimination refers to the reduction to zero of the *regional* incidence of an infectious disease; in the case of elimination, importation of infection from other regions of the world is possible, and so control measures must be continued.[3] Polio has been eliminated from the Western Hemisphere, but not yet eradicated from the globe.

Eradication programs are of necessity global in scope. They must also be vertical in design, meaning that they focus solely on a single disease. Supporters of eradication and other vertical programs have long been at odds with those in global public health who advocate the delivery of primary health care: the provision of comprehensive health services, ideally with the active participation of the communities being served. Proponents of primary health care often argue that eradication programs, and other vertical programs, do little to address the most pressing health issues of the poor. The debate is of long standing and continues today. As far back as 1969, John Bryant criticized vertical programs because "the most serious health needs cannot be met by teams with spray guns and vaccinating syringes" (quoted in Cueto 2004, 1864). More recently, Laurie Garrett argued in *Foreign Affairs* that because the current increase in funding for global health is "directed mostly at specific high-profile diseases—rather than at public health in general—there is a grave danger that the current age of generosity could not only fall short of expectations but actually make things worse on the ground" (Garrett 2007, 14).

However, vertical programs have some major strengths: they usually have clear goals, fairly straightforward methodologies, and measurable indicators of progress. And certainly, proponents of eradication and other vertical programs would never argue against the simultaneous provision of primary health care. But in a world with somewhat limited funding and—more to the point—limited staff for health interventions in poor countries, emphasis on an eradication program in a given area may come at the expense of activities aimed at improving the general health of that population. These tradeoffs may well be worth it if the eradication program succeeds—but attempts at eradication are by nature risky.

## Eradication Programs in the Twentieth Century

Eradication programs come with a high risk of failure and a high degree of difficulty. The Polio Eradication Initiative carries the promise and the risk of this approach to public health. In the twentieth century, seven human diseases—hookworm, yellow fever, yaws, malaria, smallpox, polio, and guinea worm—were targeted with large-scale campaigns for eradication. Only one project succeeded.

The Rockefeller Foundation's Sanitary Commission launched a hookworm "eradication" program in the U.S. South in 1909.[4] Hookworm is transmitted through fecal contamination of soil; people commonly contract the parasite when they walk barefoot on contaminated ground. The project included education for doctors, teachers, and the general public, as well as revival-style meetings where people were evaluated for infection and treated, if needed, en masse. While the project reduced the burden of disease of hookworm, it did not eliminate it entirely. The treatment regimen could be dangerous and was difficult to follow, and the Sanitary Commission, while it educated Southerners on the importance of privies, did not become extensively involved in privy construction itself.[5] In fact, the goal of "eradication" was likely intended only to get people excited about the project and may never have been a real goal among Sanitary Commission leaders (Ettling 1981).

The Sanitary Commission, which worked through state boards of health, also encountered some resistance from government health leaders. "There are many who feel it is dangerous to have outside agencies initiate and direct the activities of state and municipal officials," outside evaluator Charles V. Chapin wrote about the Sanitary Commission's activities in 1915. "There is probably not a health officer who is not in constant fear that some group of over-enthusiastic, and perhaps ill-advised, reformers may not, by outside pressure, bring about a one-sided diversion of the funds of his department, perhaps to lines of work of problematical value" (quoted in Ettling 1981, 196).

Partly because such domestic resistance, John Ettling argues, "made the prospect of overseas work among submissive colonials increasingly more attractive," the Rockefeller Foundation phased out its hookworm project in the South in 1914. Through its new International Health Division, it set its sights abroad (ibid.).[6] By 1920, global hookworm eradication had become a bona fide goal of the organization (Farley 2004). Hookworm campaigns were carried out in fifty-two countries and twenty-nine islands, but eradication was never achieved (Birn and Solorzano 1999). While the burden of disease caused by hookworm was reduced in some areas, the Rockefeller International Health Division was unwilling to spend much itself on improving sanitation, preferring to focus on treatment. A number of governments, both national and colonial, resisted the International Health Division's expectation that they spend large amounts of their own money on hookworm control (Birn and Solorzano 1999; Farley 2004). Further, hookworm is an extremely difficult disease to eradicate: a recent working group on eradicable disease described hookworm as "refractory to elimination in most areas" (Figueroa 1999). By 1930, the International Health Division had abandoned hookworm eradication as a goal, though "failure was never admitted as a reason for closing down" (Farley 2004, 84).

The Rockefeller Foundation also attempted to eradicate yellow fever beginning in 1915. At the time, International Health Division planners were under the impression that yellow fever transmission was possible only in the high population densities and ecologies of coastal cities. They also thought that the mosquito *Aedes aegypti* was the disease's only vector (that is, that it was the only species that could transmit the virus from one person to another). Therefore, they believed that elimination of *Ae. aegypti* in a handful of key cities would eradicate yellow fever (Farley 2004; Gubler 2004; Lowy 1997). Their strategy of mosquito control appeared to be effective: in early 1928, nearly a year had passed without a single reported case of yellow fever in the Americas. But in 1928 and 1929, outbreaks were reported both in Rio de Janeiro and in small towns in Colombia and Venezuela (Soper 1963). Further investigation revealed that yellow fever transmission was much different than had been believed. *Ae. aegypti* was not yellow fever's only vector, and humans were not its only host: rather, there was ongoing circulation of "forest yellow fever" in other species of mosquitoes and in primates. While the International Health Division continued antimosquito activities, these new discoveries put an end to hopes of eradicating yellow fever (Lowy 1997). The optimism that had led International Health Division officials to confidently predict the end of yellow fever by the mid-1920s had proved unfounded, and Fred Soper, who worked on the project, wrote later that the early 1930s were "probably this century's low point in acceptance of the eradication concept in the prevention of communicable diseases" (Soper 1965, 857).

Enthusiasm for international eradication programs was reborn after

World War II. In the United States in those years, many felt that the major infectious diseases would soon become a thing of the past (Colgrove 2006). The postwar era was characterized by optimism about international development generally; in 1949, Harry Truman announced America's intent to use its "store of technical knowledge in order to help [the people of underdeveloped nations] realize their aspirations for a better life" (quoted in Cooper and Packard 2005, 129). The model, Truman's words make clear, was to be technical: wealthy countries would provide technological fixes for the problems of poor countries. In the mid-1950s, the promise of two of these fixes—the use of injectable penicillin against yaws and of DDT against the mosquitoes that carried malaria—was so great that the World Health Organization mounted eradication campaigns against both yaws and malaria (Henderson 1998).

The World Health Organization's malaria eradication program, launched in 1955, was the largest and most expensive eradication effort prior to polio. Two new technical breakthroughs—DDT, as well as chloroquine to treat the disease—made many confident that malaria would soon disappear. "While keeping in mind the realities one can nevertheless be confident that malaria is well on its way toward oblivion," Rockefeller Foundation malariologist Paul Russell wrote in *Man's Mastery of Malaria* in 1955. "Already as a malariologist, I feel premonitory twinges of lonesomeness, and in my own organization I am now a sort of 'last survivor'" (Russell 1955, viii).

Health planners knew that malaria's insect vectors would ultimately become resistant to DDT and decided on a time-limited push to eradicate malaria from the globe forever. The plan for the eradication program focused on widespread and intensive spraying with DDT, followed by treatment of cases with chloroquine and targeted DDT spraying when only a few cases of malaria remained (Needham and Canning 2003). Originally, the program was expected to take eight years and cost a little over $500 million (Brown 1997). Ultimately, the project lasted more than ten years and cost about $1.4 billion, a third of the WHO's operating budget during that time (Centers for Disease Control and Prevention 1993; Seytre and Shaffer 2005). But eradication proved elusive, and the WHO abandoned the project in 1969.

A number of factors led to the failure of malaria eradication. The project never reached the necessary scale in sub-Saharan Africa, where killing large numbers of mosquitoes with DDT failed to have much of an effect on malaria incidence (Needham and Canning 2003). The project placed little emphasis on research—like Paul Russell, quoted earlier, many considered malariology a science that was no longer needed—and therefore did not have sufficient information on the complexities of mosquito ecology (Brown 1997). In addition, the project was designed and carried out with little regard for the preferences or participation of local populations (Packard 1997). Many people disliked DDT's side effects and resisted having their houses sprayed (Needham and Canning 2003). Over time, as predicted, mosquitoes developed resistance to DDT. The promise of the technical fix did not materialize, and planners' initial optimism proved unfounded.

At about the same time as the malaria eradication campaigns, the World Health Organization also instituted a much smaller eradication program against yaws. A nonvenereal relative of syphilis that primarily affects children, yaws was attacked with mass campaigns treating those infected with injectable penicillin (Hackett and Guthe 1956; Walker and Hay 2001). The yaws campaigns, while they did not succeed in eradicating the disease before they were largely discontinued in 1969, reduced the prevalence of yaws by 95 percent (Asiedu et al. 2008).

Against the backdrop of the failed malaria eradication program, however, disfavor for vertical programs was growing. By the 1970s, a new model for public health that set its sights squarely on primary health care programming was coming into vogue. Accompanying the focus on primary health care was a shift in perspective away from technical quick fixes like penicillin injections toward more general "development" goals like improved hygiene. In addition, according to Kristin Harper in a July 15, 2008, letter to me, yawslike infections were identified in primates, which led many to question whether eradication of the disease was possible. Yaws control was largely integrated into fledgling primary health care programs.

There was, however, one great global eradication success: smallpox. Adopted by the World Health Assembly in 1959 under Soviet pressure, the Smallpox Eradication Program initially gained little international support, receiving about one-tenth as much funding as malaria eradication over the next five years.[7] In the mid-1960s, however, the project caught the attention of Lyndon Johnson, not least as a way to improve U.S.-Soviet relations. Funding and support for the program increased, allowing it to become truly global in scope. Through a combination of flexible leadership, a culture of experimentation and innovation, and—at times—coercive tactics, smallpox was successfully eradicated in 1978 (Greenough 1995; D. Hopkins 1983; Needham and Canning 2003; Tucker 2001).

A number of factors contributed to the success of the Smallpox Eradication Program. First of all, the smallpox vaccine was a very efficient tool, conferring immunity in just one dose and effective even *after* someone had been exposed to smallpox. Also, the leadership of the program was flexible enough to switch strategies in the middle of the campaign when it became clear that mass vaccination was not the most effective method (J. Hopkins 1989).[8] Finally, in the postcolonial context, smallpox eradication officials could use coercion when they felt it was needed.

Currently, two major eradication programs are under way, of which the largest by far is the Polio Eradication Initiative. Polio is a technically more difficult disease to eradicate than smallpox, both because the vast majority of infections are "silent" and asymptomatic and because immunity to polio requires a large number of doses of vaccine—seven or more in currently endemic countries—separated by at least a month.

There is also a project, begun in 1986 and led by the Carter Center, to eradicate guinea worm. After twenty years, this parasite remains endemic in six African countries (World Health Organization 2009). In 2007, the World Health Organization increased its attention to the program—perhaps, some people there speculated, because the organization would need a success story should polio eradication fail. The program has been making sustained progress—recently, each year has seen substantially fewer cases of guinea worm than the year before, and in 2008 there were fewer than five thousand reported cases in the world, down from an estimated millions of cases per year in the 1980s (D. Hopkins et al. 2007). Still, eradication appears unlikely by the current target date, the end of 2009.[9] Uneven commitment by health authorities in some areas, as well as uncertain security in other areas, including parts of Sudan, are ongoing challenges for the program (D. Hopkins et al. 2007; World Health Organization 2008a).

## The Feasibility Concept

Planners of eradication projects often speak of the capacity of these projects to succeed in terms of two factors: technical feasibility and operational feasibility. Technical feasibility refers to biological features of the pathogen and available vaccines or other control measures. For example, eradicating HIV is not currently technically feasible, since we have no control measures (like vaccines or treatment) that can completely stop transmission of the disease. Operational feasibility refers to the capacity to deliver the necessary interventions at the necessary scale to the populations where they are needed. The question of a project's operational feasibility is often weighed in a rather abstract sense, as if planners were living in a world free of politics and competing agendas: in general, if everyone followed directions and did exactly what they were supposed to, when they were supposed to do it, would this disease be eradicated?

The success of disease elimination in one part of the world is often cited as proof that eradication is both operationally and technically feasible. For example, that polio was eliminated from Brazil is often offered as proof of the operational feasibility of eradicating polio worldwide. This type of analysis allows the political, economic, and other differences between Brazil and other countries to be sidelined. Similarly, when malaria's mosquito vector *A. gambiae* was eliminated from Brazil in 1940, the success was cited as proof that malaria eradication was technically feasible, though in fact the ecologies of the malaria parasite and its vector, including the impact of DDT spraying on transmission, varied widely in different parts of the world (Coggeshall 1944; Macdonald 1965; Needham and Canning 2003; Peter Brown, personal communication, 2008).

When people remember failed eradication programs, they often emphasize the technical reasons for their failure, such as anopheles mosquito resistance to DDT. Attributing failures to biological and epidemiological features of a targeted disease can lead to the conclusion that other targets for eradication—diseases with different biologies and modes of transmission—will not face similar difficulties. This approach contributes to optimism about eradication.

Political, economic, and cultural factors, including those that affect the global health institutions implementing eradication projects, are less often mentioned in the public health literature. Randall Packard has argued, however, that these factors contributed in major ways to the failure of malaria eradication. The malaria eradication program was launched in a climate of postwar optimism; its planners had faith in technology and its potential and believed that when problems arose, technical solutions to them would be found (Brown 1997; Packard 1997). However, their faith in technology and consequent lack of attention to social factors proved costly: Packard argues that a "constellation of technical, organizational, and financial obstacles hampered efforts at malaria eradication" (Packard 1997, 280; Packard and Brown 1997).

In the case of polio eradication, there is widespread agreement that the factors making eradication difficult are organizational, not technical. As Dr. Margaret Chan, director-general of the World Health Organization, told a meeting of donors and government representatives in Geneva: "There are no significant scientific or technical barriers to polio eradication. The problems we face are largely operational and financial" (Chan 2007a). This rhetoric of technical feasibility is echoed in numerous official Polio Eradication Initiative documents (e.g., World Health Organization 2001a, 2002, 2003, 2005b). Interestingly, in concert with admissions that operational issues are the ones hobbling polio eradication, planners continue to insist on the operational feasibility of polio eradication—asserting that it is *theoretically* possible.

Perhaps because of this framing of the issue, despite widespread agreement that organizational barriers are paramount, the Polio Eradication Initiative has conducted little research on organizational factors and does not discuss organizational issues in depth in its strategic plans. This lack is largely due to the training of people running the Initiative at the global level—virologists, epidemiologists, and doctors who see themselves as *technical* experts. A description of the nature of the organizational problems in the Polio Eradication Initiative, as well as exploration of the importance of formal discussion and planning regarding organizational and political factors and the provision of some tools for doing so, are central goals of this book. Here, the important concept to note is that "feasible" in eradication policy means *possible*; it does not necessarily mean *probable*.

## Costs and Benefits

In concert with the rhetoric of feasibility and ideological arguments about eradication as the ultimate in public health, economic cost-benefit analysis is used as an argument for implementing eradication programs in preference to other types of public health programs (e.g., Barrett 2004). Ideally, after a successful eradication program, control measures that would otherwise continue indefinitely can end.[10] Thus the financial savings to be gained posteradication go on, at least in theory, in perpetuity. The savings that the United States alone realized as a result of the success of smallpox eradication are considerable—it recoups its $30 million investment every twenty-six days in saved vaccination costs. Such savings are often cited in favor of the strategy of eradication (Centers for Disease Control and Prevention 1993).

Polio has become a priority disease precisely because it is, at least in theory, eradicable. A World Health Organization document explained that polio had been chosen as the theme of World Health Day 1995 because "polio is one of only a handful of diseases that can not only be prevented but eradicated as well" (World Health Organization 1995a, 6).

A series of cost-benefit analyses have backed arguments for polio eradication as a strategy throughout the course of the Polio Eradication Initiative (Bart, Foulds, and Patriarca 1996; Khan and Ehreth 2003; McFarland 1995; Sangrujee, Caceres, and Cochi 2004; World Health Organization 1992). Ted Turner predicted in 2000 that "once polio is eradicated and we can stop immunizing children against this scourge, the world will save

U.S. $1.5 billion dollars every year in immunization costs. Investing in polio eradication now is just good business" (UNICEF 2000). While polio eradication has already cost more than six times original estimates, it continues to look like an attractive option in cost-benefit analyses (Thompson and Tebbens 2007).

What such analyses never take into account is the possibility that a given eradication program will fail. This is a crucial omission, because eradication programs are extraordinarily expensive. The costs of stopping disease transmission in the world's hardest-to-reach populations are significant. In the case of failure, disease will likely return to these difficult areas, and hard-won gains will be lost. Thus even experts committed to the ideal of eradication speak of the "potentially enormous cost of failure" (Dowdle 1999). Eradication is a high-risk, high-gain strategy.

Because of the enormous investment required and the specter of the loss of that investment should they fail, eradication programs, once started, are difficult to stop. Polio eradication planners, in a sort of scare tactic, often speak of polio's resurgence should eradication be abandoned as a strategy. The Global Polio Eradication Initiative's 2006 annual report warns: "The alternative is unacceptable: hundreds of thousands of children would again be paralyzed by this disease over the coming years, and billions of dollars would be spent on outbreak response activities, rehabilitation/treatment costs, and associated loss of economic productivity" (World Health Organization 2007a). Beyond financial issues, polio eradication leaders warn of other fallout should the project fail. Bruce Aylward, the head of the program at WHO, said: "We have an opportunity to have an incredibly motivated health force with a great success stuck under its belt move out in search of other great challenges. Imagine the death to that motivation if we are not successful" (Thigpen 2004).

The problem is that continued funding does not ensure success of the program. Continued expenditure and effort on attempts to achieve eradication could be pouring good money (and work) after bad. Technical feasibility notwithstanding, the achievement of polio eradication is far from certain. Thus, a belief in polio eradication as a strategy is just that—a belief. This element of faith explains why religious language proves particularly apt in describing attitudes toward eradication. For example, one woman who had previously worked on polio eradication referred to its leaders as "true believers" and to herself as an "agnostic."[11] Similarly, WHO representatives exhort donors to "have faith." The tension between eradication believers and unbelievers (or, more precisely, believers in other strategies) in global health has a profound effect on the policy and rhetoric of eradication programs.

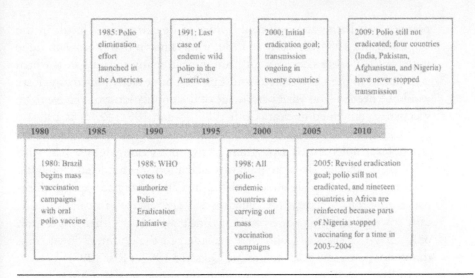

**Figure 1. Polio Eradication Initiative timeline**

## A Brief History of Polio Eradication

While eradication as a strategy was "rehabilitated" by the success of smallpox eradication in 1978 (Aylward, Hennesey, et al. 2000, 1516; Horstmann 1984), that year also marked the landmark conference in Alma-Ata promoting the concept of primary health care. Primary health care had its own cadre of true believers, not least among them Halfdan Mahler, then director-general of WHO. Mahler is reported to have said that, the success of smallpox notwithstanding, "never again would such a vertical program be promoted by the World Health Organization" (de Quadros 1997b, 183). In the mid-1980s, the status of eradication as a strategy was in question. Even D. A. Henderson, instrumental in smallpox eradication, argued that "immunization services . . . are best delivered along with other services needed by children during their first year of life and by pregnant women—the persons who constitute the priority groups for primary health care services in the developing world" (Henderson 1984, S477). In contrast to this ideal of providing immunization against a variety of diseases in the context of more comprehensive health care, polio eradication necessitated enormous mass vaccination campaigns focused solely on polio. [12]

Nor was there consensus on the technical feasibility of polio eradication. While many, notably Albert Sabin, the developer of oral polio vaccine (OPV), argued that mass vaccination could lead to eradication, others pointed out that eradication could prove to be extremely difficult in the tropics (Sabin 1984). As early as 1984, it was known that more than three doses of OPV were necessary for immunity in many tropical areas (three is sufficient in the United States and Europe); but exactly how many doses would be needed, and what percentage of the population would have to be vaccinated, remained unclear (Chin 1984; Jordan 1984; Robbins 1984).

In 1980, Brazil, troubled by polio outbreaks in several wealthy southern states, implemented a program of two mass campaigns a year with OPV (Risi 1997).[13] This program of vaccination was modeled loosely on mass campaigns implemented in 1962 in Cuba that had rapidly eliminated polio on the island (de Quadros 1992).[14] These campaigns drastically lowered the polio case count in Brazil—by 1983, their third year, only forty-five cases of polio were recorded in the country, down from thousands just a few years before (de Quadros 1997a; Risi 1997).[15]

In Brazil, as in much of the world, many supporters of primary health care were initially opposed to such efforts, which they feared would detract attention from the need to build stronger health systems. But supporters of the project argued that the successful polio vaccination campaigns in Brazil served to increase public awareness of, and support for, vaccination more generally, and thus actually strengthened primary health care (Hampton 2009). "The polio eradication effort was a key tool in implementing other immunization-related public health activities in Brazil," one man who worked in planning and implementing polio campaigns and surveillance there argued. "Public and political recognition insured a high priority for vaccination practices, disease surveillance and laboratory support. The national vaccination days soon became an operational vehicle for increasing coverage of other vaccines" (Risi 1997, 179). Such arguments were instrumental in convincing people committed to primary health care to support mass vaccination campaigns against polio.

Brazil's program was widely cited as illustrating the feasibility of polio elimination in large, poor countries. Ciro de Quadros wrote in 1997 that Brazil's experience "demonstrates that it is logistically possible to implement this strategy in a large developing country" (de Quadros 1997a, 126). Eliding the political, economic, climactic, and social differences among "large developing countries," the experience in Brazil was commonly cited as proof that polio could be eliminated *anywhere*.

In 1981, the Pan American Health Organization (PAHO) and the Fogarty International Center of the U.S. National Institutes of Health held a conference on polio and concluded that elimination of the disease in the Western Hemisphere was technically feasible. In 1984, Ciro de Quadros, the committed and by all accounts charismatic man who would become the leader of the polio elimination effort in the Americas, met with James Grant, then executive director of UNICEF. With its focus on children, UNICEF was already committed to routine childhood immunization; de Quadros convinced Grant that polio could be a "banner disease" for immunizations in general (de Quadros 1997b, 185).[16]

Rotary International also joined the effort. Rotary had first become involved in polio immunization in 1979, when the organization funded the vaccination of six million children in the Philippines.[17] Over the next five years, Rotary organized campaigns in five more countries. Such large international service projects, requiring the commitment and participation of many clubs, were new ground for Rotary. They were part of an effort to tie its diverse worldwide membership together (Hampton 2009; Pigman 2005).[18] As William Sergeant, chair of Rotary's PolioPlus program for many years, explained:

> Until 1978, Rotary clubs acted individually in their communities. Then we decided to do something that would involve all members worldwide, something important that clubs couldn't do alone. The eradication of a disease corresponded to our will to do something together, and gradually we reached the conclusion that the disease should be polio. Our choice had a great deal to do with the fact that polio affects little people, the most innocent members of society. We still had Rotary leaders who remembered the terribly crippling effects of polio in the U.S. (Seytre and Shaffer 2005, 104–105)

In 1982, Rotary committed to the goal of "immunizing all the world's children against polio." Having never attempted such a project, Rotary was perhaps overoptimistic about the ease with which it would be achieved. As a prominent Rotarian later commented: "If we had realized all the complexity, that decision would never have been made" (Pigman 2005, 32).

In 1984, Albert Sabin approached Rotary looking for support for the polio elimination effort in the Americas.[19] Rotary pledged $120 million for vaccines, and raised over $200 million for the effort in less than two years (de Quadros 1997b; Hampton 2009).[20] Rotary's involvement was key to securing both funding and political commitment for the nascent project. With Rotary's support, USAID also joined the effort.

This collaboration between PAHO, UNICEF, Rotary, and USAID was the first major international partnership of UN, bilateral, and private agencies in the health sector, and a major change from the more insular way in which these agencies had traditionally worked. All these agencies said that they supported mass polio immunization campaigns as a way to increase immunization rates in general—as a way of *furthering* primary health care (Hampton 2009). Rotary's official literature explained that its wing of the program was named PolioPlus,

> in recognition that control of polio is only one sector of the battle to improve child health, and that PolioPlus should support and complement the goals of the Expanded Programme on Immunization (EPI) of WHO. Furthermore, it is recognized that EPI itself is part of a broader primary health care strategy to improve child health. (Rotary Foundation 1985, 187)[21]

There was widespread popular support for polio immunization in the Americas (Hampton 2009), and the project went well. By 1987, all polio-endemic countries in the Americas were carrying out mass vaccination campaigns (de Quadros and Henderson 1993). These campaigns had an impact: by 1989, even with increased surveillance quality, the number of cases of polio was down to 128 in the Americas, compared to 930 just three years before (de Quadros 1992).

The partners in the elimination effort in the Americas soon set their sights on a more ambitious goal: the global eradication of polio. A number of advocates, including Ciro de Quadros and the smallpox veteran Bill Foege, claimed that "global eradication could be achieved as early as 1995" (Hinman et al. 1987, 835). At a conference in Taillores, France, in March 1988, Halfdan Mahler, the director-general of WHO, was convinced that the eradication of polio could strengthen routine immunization provision in particular and health services in general and agreed to support the strategy of polio eradication (Aylward, Acharya, and England 2003; de Quadros 1997b).[22]

At the World Health Assembly two months later, Mahler urged member states to agree to support the goal of polio eradication:

> Of course I could add [to smallpox eradication] many more success stories that have been initiated by your WHO. Who would have thought this among you the cynics and the skeptics? When you the World Health Assembly said we should be immunizing all the world's children by 1990 against the major killers of childhood diseases, I do not think anybody believed we should get anywhere. . . . Indeed, I would like to challenge you. On the basis of these results, what about having the guts

to suggest that we should eradicate poliomyelitis from spaceship Earth by the year 2000? I think we should, I think it is do-able and therefore there is not any excuse for not trying, and trying very hard, to do it. (Mahler 1988)

The 166 members of the World Health Assembly unanimously voted to undertake the eradication of polio as an "appropriate gift, along with the eradication of smallpox, from the twentieth to the twenty-first century" (World Health Assembly 1988). The objective was to achieve polio eradication by the year 2000.

The choice to take on eradication was indeed gutsy, as even Brazil, the country whose experience was most often cited as proof that polio eradication could be achieved, did not see its last case of polio until 1989, a year later. The structure of the Global Polio Eradication Initiative was based on that developed by Ciro de Quadros for the Americas. In the Americas, de Quadros had instituted a system which included: (1) mass campaigns of oral polio vaccine held twice a year at fixed points to which parents brought children under five; (2) door-to-door mop-up campaigns in areas of persistent transmission; (3) labs to determine whether cases of paralysis were in fact due to polio; and (4) "technical advisory groups" of international experts to advise national governments on policy. This basic structure was adopted by the global campaign and continued throughout most of the 1990s. The strategy of polio eradication, then and now, was to achieve as high a coverage as possible in children under five with mass campaigns of oral polio vaccine, while ideally maintaining high routine immunization coverage.[23] The same partners in the elimination campaign in the Americas—UNICEF, Rotary, CDC, and the WHO (PAHO in the Americas)—were the spearheading partners of the global project. UNICEF formally committed to global polio eradication at the World Summit for Children in 1991.

Despite its unanimous adoption by the World Health Assembly and the support of a broad range of partners, global polio eradication got off to a slow start. Many in WHO were still skeptical of eradication as a strategy and of polio eradication in particular (Needham and Canning 2003). Other global priorities, including the emerging HIV/AIDS pandemic, took precedence over polio. International promotion of polio eradication was limited, funding was insufficient, and research was not ramped up to the necessary levels (Aylward and Heymann 2005; World Health Organization 1990). As of 1993, the most highly polio-endemic countries in South Asia and sub-Saharan Africa were conducting neither surveillance nor mass campaigns (Ward and Hull 1995). Pakistan, India, and Bangladesh accounted for around 75 percent of worldwide polio cases in early 1994 (Davey 1997); none of them had yet implemented a single mass campaign.[24]

However, the Americas saw their last case of endemic polio—in Peru—in 1991, and in 1993, China began the largest-scale activities thus far, immunizing eighty-three million children in a single round and achieving elimination by 1995 (Davey 1997).[25] These events helped provide the impetus for scaling up polio eradication in the mid to late 1990s, a process that has only intensified since. In 1996, Nelson Mandela launched the Kick Polio Out of Africa campaign, and twenty-eight African countries began immunization activities over the next three years. Also in 1996, U.S. contributions to polio eradication quadrupled after Rotarians testified to Congress on its importance; in 1997, the United States donated $72 million to polio eradication (World Health Organization 1997).[26] Global expenditures increased rapidly, from well under $100 million in 1995 to about $200 million in 1997. The scale of activities reached impressive levels fairly quickly: in 1995, 300 million children, nearly half the world's under-five population, were immunized against polio. In 1996, the number reached 420 million; and in 2000, 600 million children received OPV. However, in interviews with me and with others (e.g., Seytre and Shaffer 2005, 117), polio planners have conceded that given the late start to eradication activities in the highest-transmission countries, the goal of eradication by 2000 was probably never realistic. In fact, all endemic countries did not begin mass campaigns until 1988, and house-to-house campaigns and adequate surveillance were not present in all parts of the world until 2000 itself (World Health Organization 2001b). In Pakistan, the intensification of activities, which involved the transition from conducting fixed-point campaigns (i.e., vaccinating children at a central location) to house-to-house campaigns (in which each home in the nation is visited) was not implemented until 1999.

In 2000, with transmission ongoing in around twenty countries, the end date for the Polio Eradication Initiative was pushed back to 2005, the hundredth anniversary of Rotary. Ted Turner, Kofi Annan, and Mia Farrow were present at the United Nations' New York Visitor's Center for the unveiling of a giant clock that counted down the seconds until 2005. As house-to-house campaigns and improved surveillance were implemented in endemic countries, the yearly budget increased again, to around $400 million. Progress continued until 2003, when just 784 cases of polio were reported in six endemic countries (down from an estimated hundreds of thousands of cases per year in the late 1980s). In 2004, the budget was set at nearly $700 million a year, with the aim of eliminating the last few cases. The number of campaigns rose to as many as eight a year in endemic areas, each requiring huge numbers of people to implement vaccination efforts. In Pakistan, a single nationwide campaign employs 200,000 workers to vaccinate around 30 million children; in India, 2.3 million workers vaccinate nearly 170 million children under five in a national campaign.

But despite frequent and carefully planned large-scale campaigns, polio transmission continues in Pakistan, India, Afghanistan, and Nigeria. The 2005 deadline passed, with WHO officials claiming each year that this will be the last. The increasing case count is in part due to suspension of vaccination in parts of Nigeria in 2003 because of concerns that mass administration of OPV was part of a Western plot to harm Nigerians. By the time polio vaccination was resumed in all of Nigeria in 2004, the northern states of the country were heavily infected and the virus had spread to fourteen previously polio-free countries (World Health Organization 2005a). However, poliovirus circulation has also stubbornly persisted in

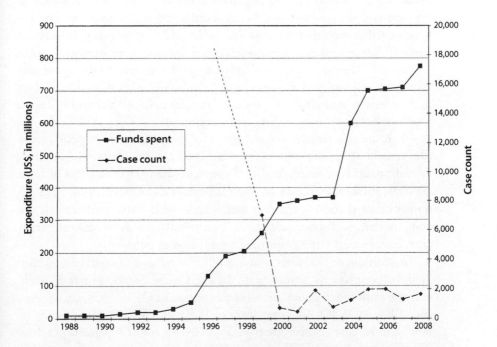

**Figure 2. The Polio Eradication Initiative's yearly expenditure and estimate of polio cases globally. (Good surveillance was not yet in place prior to 1999; however, in 1993 the WHO estimated that there were about 100,000 cases of polio globally [Rafei 1995].)**

Afghanistan, Pakistan, and India, countries where immunization activities were never suspended.

Because of the huge amount of money necessary to carry out polio eradication in these late stages of the program, and donors' growing skepticism about the possibility of polio eradication, funding crises are ongoing. Even with nearly $800 million a year, the global scale of polio eradication means that lack of funds sometimes limits eradication activities in Pakistan to the highest-risk areas of the country only.

## The Culture of Optimism

Polio eradication's true believers have not given up the fight. In February 2007, WHO held a conference in Geneva to rally donors and endemic-country governments. Admitting that "these last 4 countries have been 'stuck' at 500–1500 cases/year, in the same geographic areas," WHO and its partner agencies offered donors "new approaches in each of the 4 endemic areas" (World Health Organization et al. 2007). In Pakistan and Afghanistan, they touted "new cross-border strategies" as an innovative approach that would end transmission. In addition to being objectively false—Pakistan and Afghanistan have had "cross-border strategies" since 1998—this "new solution" to Pakistan's problems overlooks significant centers of ongoing transmission *not* on the border with Afghanistan. But such an extremely bullish take on the future of polio eradication has been a hallmark of the program since its inception.

There are at least two major reasons for the persistence of polio in the four remaining endemic countries. One is epidemiological. Polio is transmitted primarily through fecal-oral contact (when water supplies or food are contaminated with human waste). Polio is also a heat-loving virus, so transmission is most intense in warm areas with poor sanitation. India and Pakistan, with poor sanitation, high population densities, and warm climates, are ideal settings for the transmission of poliovirus.

In addition, the number of doses of OPV needed to confer immunity in these populations is very high. In the United States, nearly all children are immune to poliovirus after three doses of OPV (McBean, Thoms, and Albrecht 1988). In some areas of India, in contrast, the efficacy of oral polio vaccine against one type of poliovirus is just 9 percent per dose (Grassly et al. 2006).[27] This means that ten or more doses of oral polio vaccine, spaced a month apart, are necessary for population immunity in these areas. The challenge, of course, is that babies are constantly being born who must be immunized. Babies receive protection from polio from maternal antibodies for about the first six months of life. Clearly, however, it is impossible to deliver ten doses of vaccine, spaced one month apart, within the span of six months. New vaccines have recently been developed that confer immunity in fewer doses, but they have not proved to be a magic bullet in India or Pakistan.[28] The difficulty of delivering so many doses of vaccine to every child in the country is why planners in Geneva have described the situation in a few states in India as "fragile" and "dangerous."

In Pakistan, polio eradication is epidemiologically a bit easier than in these parts of India. However, Pakistan still presents a challenge. In 2006, surveillance data showed that in 93 percent of districts in Pakistan, the median number of OPV doses that children under five had received was more than 7; it was more than three in 99 percent of districts.[29] Put simply, if immunity to polio in Pakistan required, as in the United States, only three doses of vaccine, poliovirus would have already been eliminated in Pakistan.

That said, that polio has been eliminated from the most epidemiologically difficult areas of Pakistan illustrates that the problems the Polio Eradication Initiative faces are not purely epidemiological. They are also organizational and political. A detailed exploration of these issues is the work of other chapters in this book. Here it will suffice to say that in Pakistan, a country being pulled apart at the seams by power struggles among parties as diverse as the army, political parties, lawyers' associations, the United States, and the Taliban, polio eradication is not and will not in the near future become a political priority.

Neither of these issues—difficult disease ecology in tropical countries with high population density and the problem of political indifference—was unforeseeable in early planning for polio eradication. Many concerned parties discussed them both well before 1988. That oral polio vaccine in India did not produce levels of immunity comparable to that in industrialized countries was observed in the 1970s and discussed in mid-1980s conferences on the feasibility of eradication (John 1984). As discussed earlier, researchers also knew in the mid-1980s that polio eradication would be epidemiologically difficult in the tropics, although precisely how many doses of OPV would be needed to confer population immunity in, for example, India was not clearly established. Similarly, that not every country in the world has embraced polio eradication as a top priority simultaneously should hardly come as a surprise to seasoned global health planners. In short, the problems that polio eradication is currently facing were predictable.

However, from 1988 forward, the threats these issues posed to the future of eradication were consistently minimized, even ignored. Instead, an optimistic stream of rhetoric and planning proceeded as if these difficulties did not exist. To be fair, no one knew just how serious they would become, but the rhetoric of polio eradication in the mid-1990s seems willfully naïve in retrospect. For example, in 1993, planners believed that if all endemic countries conducted two mass campaigns per year from fixed points by 1995, supplemented with house-to-house mop-up activities twice per year in stubborn areas by 1997, polio would be eradicated by the year 2000 (Ward et al. 1993). Worldwide, countries were not sufficiently enthused about polio eradication to adopt it on this schedule, but even if they had, current experience shows that this schedule of immunizations would have been woefully inadequate to interrupt transmission in places like India and Pakistan.

Projections of the cost, scale, and duration of the project reflect just how optimistic planners have been over the course of polio eradication. The end date for the project, in Pakistan and globally, has always been the topic of highly optimistic speculation and planning:

1987    "Global eradication could be achieved as early as 1995" (Hinman et al. 1987, 835).

1994    It was assumed polio eradication could be achieved in Pakistan in "two to three years" (CDC official, interview, Atlanta).

1995    "Can polio be eradicated on target by the year 2000? Yes, it can" (World Health Organization 1995b).

1998    "It is evident that wild poliovirus transmission worldwide can be interrupted by the end of the year 2000 or shortly thereafter, and that global eradication can be certified by the target date of 2005, provided the resources needed for both efforts are rapidly made available" (World Health Organization 1998a).[30]

2001    "The TAG reaffirms that it is epidemiologically feasible to eradicate wild poliovirus from Pakistan by the end of 2002. The next six months are the most critical period in the effort to eradicate polio from Pakistan" (Technical Advisory Groups on Polio Eradication in Afghanistan and Pakistan 2001, 3).

2004    "God willing, with our collective support, we will add another chapter of glory to the history of public health and mankind by eradicating poliomyelitis this year" (Muhammad Nasir Khan, Minister of Health, Pakistan [Khan 2004]).

2005    "The consultation has concluded that Pakistan can stop WPV [wild poliovirus] transmission in 2005" (World Health Organization 2005c).

2006    "I am still very hopeful that an aggressive approach will stop
        transmission in Pakistan in 2006" (WHO official, interview,
        Geneva).
2007    "The remaining period of 2007 presents an exceptional and
        unprecedented opportunity to interrupt wild poliovirus
        transmission in the last remaining transmission zones of
        Afghanistan and Pakistan" (Technical Advisory Groups on
        Polio Eradication in Afghanistan and in Pakistan 2007, 1).

Repeated disappointments have not quelled organizational optimism.
When asked about prospects for the future, a World Health Organization
official told me in 2007: "A few small different things happening and we
could have finished two years ago." He said that circulation of poliovirus
was "tenuous" and added: "I think this is going to be a very good year for
us."

Tied to optimism about the end date for polio eradication is optimism
about the amount of funding necessary to see the program to completion.
In 1988, the estimate for total program costs for polio eradication was
$150 million for 1988 to 2000 (World Health Organization 1988). By
1995, that estimate had risen to $800 million (Ward and Hull 1995). By
1996, with the intensification of activities, the figure was raised to $2.5
billion (World Health Organization 1996). As of the end of 2008, about
$7 billion had already been spent on polio eradication, and if history is
any indication, future expenditures will exceed the approximately $2 bil-
lion currently budgeted.

Nor will polio eradication efforts end with the last case. Circulating
vaccine virus from oral polio vaccine has the potential to become virulent and cause outbreaks of paralytic polio.[31] The first such outbreak, in
Hispaniola in 2000, caused twenty-one cases of paralysis; subsequent outbreaks occurred on an island off Java in 2005, causing forty-six cases, and
in Nigeria in 2007 (Kew et al. 2002; Pallansch and Sandhu 2006; Roberts 2007). Some immunocompromised individuals continue to excrete
vaccine virus for many years after being vaccinated, and viruses in such
individuals have been documented to develop virulence (Bellmunt et al.
1999). Thus, even the last case of wild polio will likely be followed by additional cases or outbreaks of polio from vaccine-derived poliovirus.

The phenomenon of optimistic projections succeeded by difficult realities is not unique to the Polio Eradication Initiative. In 1967, Albert
Hirschman described what he called the phenomenon of the "hiding
hand" in development projects. Hirschman believed that potential prob-

lems were often underestimated in the planning stages of a development project, but that when such problems arose creative solutions were usually found—solutions that in many cases resulted in superior projects. If these problems had been foreseen at the start of the project, Hirschman suggests, most of these projects would never have been funded, but by and large they work, and work well. While hiding costs and exaggerating benefits can lead to "disaster," Hirschman argues, they can also lead to "opportunity." Hirschman believes that the hiding-hand phenomenon happens most often in projects like the Polio Eradication Initiative, where planners are bound to the project by the time problems arise, in the sense of having spent large amounts of "money, time and energy and having committed their prestige" (Hirschman 1967, 30, 20).

Hirschman's astute analysis illustrates that the culture of optimism is not peculiar to polio eradication but shared by a wide range of development projects. But optimism in polio eradication, and perhaps in other development projects as well, is not just a phenomenon or a technique—it is a culture. By this I mean that optimism in polio eradication is not just a calculated strategy for acquiring and maintaining the support necessary to implement such a large-scale project (though it is that sometimes), but a socially shared symbol system that provides a collective language and a collective identity.

I talked to a woman who had worked with the Polio Eradication Initiative in the mid-1990s and was involved in some projections that, in retrospect, are ridiculously optimistic. I initially found this puzzling, as she is a very smart woman. She no longer works within polio eradication and is currently not highly optimistic about its prospects. When I asked about the projections she had made, she attributed the optimism at least in part to the work's occurring "within the bowels of WHO. I was sitting there; . . . you get caught up in the group and you believe the things the epidemiologists say and the technical folks say." Optimism in polio eradication is a social phenomenon.

While nearly all planners for polio eradication could be accurately described as optimistic, the partner organization for which people work affects their degree of optimism. The WHO, for example, is often described as a more optimistic place than the CDC. One person who had worked with both agencies told me that at the CDC "there is optimism but there's also . . . a kind of . . . reality optimism," meaning that the CDC was not as wildly optimistic as WHO. A CDC employee said that "WHO has always erred on the side of optimism," while CDC tends to think "realism would be better" and "doesn't like B.S." Optimism in polio eradication is cultural, and it has concrete implications.

## Structure: The Optimists and the Pakistani Government

The cultures of CDC and WHO, like all cultures, are based in social organization and economics. An outline of the structure of the Polio Eradication Initiative is key to understanding both its trajectory and its cultures. Polio eradication policy and fund-raising are run by the four spearheading partners of the Initiative: Rotary, WHO, CDC, and UNICEF. Rotary's primary work is raising funds and advocating for the project, both through its members and through the leverage it is able to exert on governments. The U.S. government is the single largest donor to polio eradication, having given over $1 billion thus far, in no small part because of Rotary lobbying. WHO is perhaps the central agency, responsible for providing policy and staff for implementation of eradication campaigns. WHO is also the agency most responsible for speaking to donors about polio eradication, a fact likely not unconnected to its highly optimistic outlook. CDC gives technical support, primarily in the areas of laboratory development and surveillance. UNICEF is responsible for vaccine logistics and for "social mobilization"—advertising and activities aimed at motivating people in countries with campaigns to ensure that children are immunized. While disagreements between the four spearheading agencies do occur, in general the partnership and the division of labor among the agencies work fairly well. People at one agency may at times disagree with the way another agency carries out its mandates, but in general it is accepted that polio eradication is too large a project for any one agency to carry out on its own, and the involvement of the other partners is seen as necessary.

The CDC and Rotary are also donors to polio eradication, providing funds of their own. The majority of funding, though, comes from other donors who are not involved in day-to-day administration of polio eradication but who ultimately determine whether the program will continue. As people at WHO headquarters in Geneva spoke about spinning information positively "for the donors," this setup does contribute to the culture of optimism. Major donors to polio eradication include USAID, the governments of the United Kingdom and Japan, the Gates Foundation, and the World Bank. Donors have, over the past five years or so, consistently been on the receiving end of the Polio Eradication Initiative's optimistic projections, and they are acutely aware that polio eradication is more difficult than they were initially led to believe. Some, like JICA (the Japanese bilateral aid agency) in Pakistan, have quietly begun shifting funds to other projects. Others, like DFID (the United Kingdom's agency) in Pakistan, say that they "have not lost faith yet" but view the Polio Eradication Initiative's projections with an increasingly skeptical eye. Thus far,

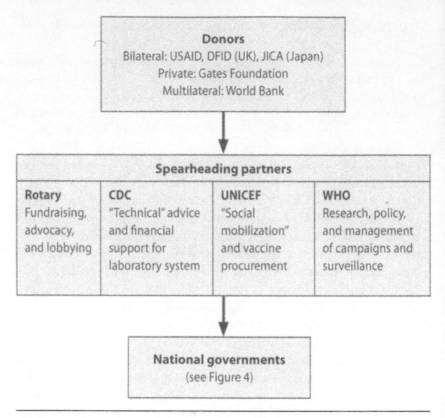

**Figure 3. The Polio Eradication Initiative at the global level**

rising skepticism in donor agencies seems only to have led the WHO and its partners to increase the volume of their optimistic statements.

The structure of the Polio Eradication Initiative in Pakistan reflects the ideals currently in vogue in global public health of partnership and collaboration between international agencies and national governments. Officially, polio eradication is a government program in the country where it is being carried out. The implementation of polio eradication campaigns is the responsibility of the government of the country and the district where campaigns are taking place. Employees of international agencies like WHO are supposed to provide support to the government. There are about forty-five international employees of WHO and UNICEF in Pakistan. In addition, WHO alone employs more than 120 drivers and an additional 200 Pakistani nationals. Pakistan has the highest concentration of national and international WHO employees working on polio eradication of any country in the world.[32] This being the case, however, several hun-

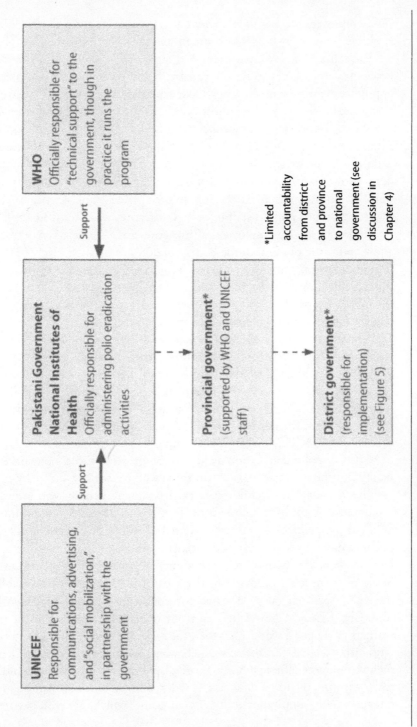

**UNICEF**

Responsible for communications, advertising, and "social mobilization," in partnership with the government

**WHO**

Officially responsible for "technical support" to the government, though in practice it runs the program

Support

Support

**Pakistani Government National Institutes of Health**

Officially responsible for administering polio eradication activities

**Provincial government***

(supported by WHO and UNICEF staff)

**District government***

(responsible for implementation)

(see Figure 5)

*Limited accountability from district and province to national government (see discussion in Chapter 4)

**Figure 4. The Polio Eradication Initiative at the national level: Islamabad**

dred employees are hardly sufficient to vaccinate thirty million children multiple times every year. Government employees must do that.

Pakistan's Health Department is a large and highly political bureaucracy. At the national level, it is run by the minister of health, a political appointee who may or may not have expertise in the area of health and who is not involved in the project on a day-to-day basis (I saw the minister of health only once in months of working at the national offices). The minister's subordinate, the head of the Expanded Programme of Immunization, is a doctor who is, at least in theory, responsible for the national administration of polio eradication activities, as well as the administration of other routine immunizations for children. The lack of practical involvement of this man and his staff in polio eradication was a source of constant frustration to WHO employees. While government officials may trot out a few optimistic phrases for the benefit of donors and high-level WHO officials, in general, employees of the Pakistani government are realists about polio eradication's prospects.

At the district level, all government health activities, including polio eradication, fall under the supervision of the executive director of health (EDO) of a district. The EDO is somewhat accountable to the government health department at the provincial level, and only weakly accountable at the national level. He can, however, be fired by the *nazim*, the elected official, of the district in which he works. Thus the EDO is of necessity a part of the political machine at the district level, has only weak responsibility to the national health office, and has no responsibility at all to WHO or UNICEF. Most WHO employees see the active participation of EDOs in polio eradication as key to the project's success but have difficulty putting effective pressure on those who resist their authority.

The vaccination of children is carried out by people who are called "volunteers" in the official literature. They are, in Pakistan, not volunteers. While the appellation "volunteer" is used to justify paying them only two dollars a day for the five days a campaign lasts, polio eradication's ground-level workers are, with a few exceptions, impoverished and disgruntled. Some of them are employees of the Health Department, answerable to the EDO for their salary not just for polio but for their other work as well. The EDO, if he wishes, can put considerable pressure on these workers to do good work. However, the scale of polio eradication necessitates hiring a large number of workers who are not regular Health Department employees. These volunteers are displeased about their pay and not really accountable to anyone, as the worst punishment that can be meted out to them is simply not to hire them again (which, at these pay levels, few see as a huge loss). Some of them do truly excellent work. Others do not.

The culture of optimism in polio eradication goes beyond eradication's success and cost to encompass the methods used to carry it out. The spearheading partners, as well as the donors, are part of larger cultures of global health and development that heavily value concepts of collaboration, participation, and ownership by host governments. These concepts inform polio eradication policy in direct ways. As polio eradication is a government project in countries where it is being implemented, WHO and UNICEF are, on paper, limited to advisory roles. In countries like China, whose government embraced the project of polio eradication and had the power and authority to carry it out, this approach works. In a place like Pakistan, where other extremely pressing issues prevent polio from becoming a political priority, and where the central government has only weak

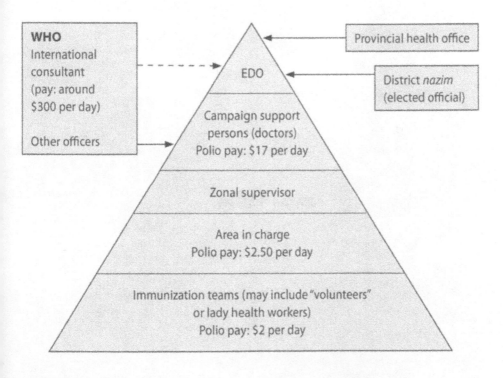

**Figure 5. The Polio Eradication Initiative at the district level**

control over peripheral districts and territories, it has not worked very well. But the culture of optimism and the global ideal of collaboration prevent these issues from being openly discussed in policy meetings. Rather, ever more optimistic though objectively false statements that "the Head of Government is now directly engaged in completing polio eradication" (World Health Organization et al. 2007) characterize rhetoric at the international level.

At the ground level, WHO employees use a number of techniques to attempt to pressure government officials into action while upholding the ideals of collaboration and support. The next chapter is a description of a situation where these fictions broke down. It illustrates the reach and limits of UN power, and the limited but nonetheless significant ability of district governments to resist international mandates.

## The Moving Target

Nasrin lives in a small thatch compound on the edge of a
settled neighborhood on the outskirts of Kaifabad. I am
at her house because her family is seminomadic, raising
goats for a living. What polio eradication planners call
"mobile populations" appear to be spreading poliovirus
across Pakistan and Afghanistan. I want to ask her about
the immunization status of her children and her experiences
with the polio immunization campaigns.

The dirt floors in her thatch hut and in the adjacent
courtyard fenced off with thatch have been vigorously
swept clean, broom marks still showing in the dirt. I sit
inside Nasrin's hut on a foam pad covered with a blanket,
with a roll pillow for my back. A small boy brings me a tall
glass mug of very sweet tea. Nasrin and her mother-in-law,
Huma, who sit and talk to me, wear the full skirts that
people in the Punjab associate with Afghanis. Nasrin wears
a heavily embroidered, handworked shirt and a gauze shawl
covered in sequins. She breastfeeds her six-month-old as we
talk, then swaddles him securely in a few pieces of cloth and
a strap and places him in a white metal cradle, her only piece
of furniture. She has a radio, and her family has managed to
rig electricity into the hut, but there is no television.

Huma, sparkling and animated, has bells braided into
her hair. Despite her very limited Urdu, she rapidly and
smilingly arranges a marriage between my one-year-old son
and her two-year-old granddaughter. Huma was born in
Afghanistan but has been in Pakistan for twenty-five years.
She spent most of her life in Waziristan, on the Pakistani
side of the border, and has been in Kaifabad for four years.
Nasrin, who speaks passable Urdu though she has never been

to school, estimates her husband sells an average of two to four goats a month for around Rs. 2,000 (about $35) apiece.

We talk about the health of Nasrin's young son and eleven-month-old nephew, a small, weak child. The women have taken him repeatedly to a nearby private clinic, which they like because the doctor there speaks their native language. This doctor (who may or may not be a doctor— unlicensed practitioners flourish in Pakistan) has given the boy a number of shots and tonics, but the boy remains "weak." I ask if any of the children in the extended family have received routine immunizations. No, Nasrin says. Why not? I ask. Was Nasrin, or someone else in the family, opposed to vaccination? "No," she says. "I don't know where they give immunizations."

Nasrin and others in her husband's extended family allow their children to be immunized for polio whenever the vaccinators come to their house—which is not every campaign. Sometimes, they say, they see the women going door-to-door at the nearby houses, but their marginal compound is not visited.

"How much are those women paid?" asks Nasrin regarding the vaccinators.

I tell her: 100 rupees (about $1.70) a day.

"That's all?" Nasrin asks. "Oh, well, then obviously they're only going to work as hard as they feel like [*apni marzi-se kām kartehein*]."

# CHAPTER 3

# Polio Eradication in Practice

I WAS THE ARBITER of the meaning of the faint brown mark on the three-year-old's fingernail. The doorway of her house, a nearly windowless brick-and-cement building sharing three of four walls with other homes, was dark, so I asked her to come out into the bright, dusty, narrow dirt street. There in the sunlight, I squatted down to look at her finger. Four people leaned over me to get a look: the lady health worker responsible for doing door-to-door polio immunization in this area, her "area in charge" or immediate supervisor, the "zonal supervisor" at a level above the area in charge, and my research assistant, Tanveer. The girl's mother, father, and uncle watched from the doorway. The area in charge was scolding the mother.

"Why are you lying to us?" he cried. "We vaccinated this child!"

"They didn't come," the father said to me. "I know, because my ad agency was working on publicity for you—the dates were the twenty-fourth through the twenty-sixth, right? And there was supposed to be Vitamin A? Nobody came to our house."

The zonal supervisor grasped the child's hand and held it up to my face. "Look at this. Obviously her finger has been marked."

I inspected the tiny, faded mark on the girl's finger. It could have been anything: a speck of nail polish, a dot of henna, or a remnant of the permanent-marker stripe that polio workers are supposed to draw on a child's finger when they give the child polio vaccine. It was impossible to tell.

I stood up. I said that I had to record the child as missed, since the parents said the child had not been immunized, workers had not marked the date of their visit to the house on the door with chalk as they were supposed to, and there was no clear mark on the child's finger.

The father stepped into the street and picked up his child. The area in charge, trying a different tack, told me he had personally visited the house multiple times but the mother was sleeping or lazy and didn't bring her children to the door.

"Tell your wife to come to the door when people come!" he told the father. "I was here three times and she just sleeps and sleeps!"

The father was admirably polite under this onslaught. I told the supervisors we needed to vaccinate these children, and they reluctantly pulled out the vaccine and the record sheets. The uncle brought out the girl's two young siblings and an infant cousin, all of whom were unvaccinated. A supervisor squeezed drops of vaccine into the children's mouths, and I marked their fingers with the permanent marker. Tanveer wrote the date, the number of children immunized, and my initials on the door with chalk.

That four children had been missed in one area meant that I would write up a report naming this a "red area," which would reflect poorly on this lady health worker, these supervisors, and this district as a whole. As we left, the supervisors tried to convince me that since they had visited the house repeatedly (both were now claiming to have come to the house), and since these were "sleeping people," the missed children shouldn't count against them. It was odd, I thought, that all this activity supposedly took place around a house with no chalk marking, as workers are supposed to mark the door of a house with chalk on each visit. I said only that I could not falsify data.

"I am a poor man," the area in charge said. "If four children are reported missed in my area, I will lose my job. I have a family to support. Please, just mark down one or two children, not four."

I squirmed. I suspected he was being overdramatic, but I couldn't be sure. He was certainly poor; I knew his salary was about a hundred dollars a month. The vaccination teams in the rest of his area had done good work. I said again that I could not falsify data. I said I would tell the executive director of health of the district that overall his work was good, that my choice of this house to survey could just have been bad luck for him, and that this mistake certainly didn't warrant firing him.

Both supervisors were angry. "Whatever you say, madam," one grumbled.

Driving home, Tanveer said to me, "Svea, if you were Pakistani, you would overlook these children for that man's sake."

"Do you think he'll really be fired?" I asked Tanveer.

"I don't know," he said.

# The Foreign Consultant

This chapter describes my participation in the spring of 2007 in a polio immunization campaign in a district I call Kaifabad, a city in the Punjab with a population of over four million. Campaigns took place over a period of about two weeks, of which eight days were filled with frenzied activity. The actual vaccination of thirty million children in Pakistan was carried out everywhere in the country over a period of only three days, with two additional days for catch-up, vaccinating children not at home when the team first visited. Finally, monitoring, or spot-checking areas to assess vaccination coverage, occurred over three days after the campaign was completed.

The campaign I describe in this chapter was the fourth I was involved in. Six months previously, I had participated in my first campaign, in another district. Then, I had assumed my participant observation would be low-key, that I would follow low-level workers around, talk to some parents, and perhaps get some interviews with higher-level district health staff. However, upon arriving in the district I was immediately thrust into the role of foreign consultant, one with a great deal of supervisory responsibility, despite the fact that at that point I had been involved in polio eradication for only two months. I rode in UN Land Cruisers, had tea with hospital directors and high-level government officials, was expected to report on the quality of work being done, and was addressed with a variety of honorifics. The experience was surreal, but I learned an extraordinary amount, and I decided that rather than try to struggle against the position in which I found myself, I would make the most of this opportunity to experience polio vaccination campaigns from the inside.

I was expected to act as a foreign consultant in all the districts I visited for several reasons. Most importantly, every other foreigner in polio eradication was in this role (and there were a lot of them in Pakistan—more than forty assigned to the country full time plus others who came and went). These included WHO foreign consultants based in Pakistan, whose salary and per diems amounted to $10,000 a month; "volunteers" from other countries sent by the CDC who did not receive a salary but had generous per diems; and international observers from Geneva. It is natural, then, that as a foreigner with ties to the WHO in Islamabad, I was immediately expected to fill this role in every district I visited. I always attempted to be clear about my status as a student and a researcher, but in truth my practice of openly sharing my observations with people at all levels of the polio eradication hierarchy made me a de facto evaluator of the districts that I visited.

My position yielded rich understandings of the nature of polio eradication campaigns in Pakistan. It also carried opportunities to advocate for the lowest-level, poorest-paid workers. However, it brought with it ethical dilemmas. On the one hand, I lost sleep over situations like the one just described, where it seemed that my actions might cause people to lose their jobs. On the other hand, I did not think that falsifying data was appropriate behavior on my part, especially since it would mean lying to people in Islamabad whose extraordinary openness and honesty made my work possible. As events unfolded, the ethical and practical prudence of my inclination to be as honest and open as possible at all times was reinforced.

## Preparing for the Campaign

Kaifabad is a dense, crowded city of several million people in the Punjab with a rapidly growing population: it doubled between the 1981 and 1998 censuses, and people continue to move to the city from rural areas. The city's edges are marked by rapid, chaotic, haphazard development; urban planning is often poor or nonexistent. According to World Bank data, only about 75 percent of the population in the city has easy access to water from a pipe or a well (though this water may not be entirely free from contamination), and only 35 percent is served by piped sewers. In most areas, open sewers run down the sides of narrow alleyways.

Near the center of the city, served by a wide road that suffers a near-perpetual traffic jam, enormous bazaars made up of hundreds of tiny shops stretch for blocks. In some of the older parts of the city, multiple families live in crowded houses served by alleyways so narrow that people on small motorcycles must navigate carefully. In wealthy areas, enormous gated bungalows are shaded by trees and separated by spacious walled yards.

Only about half the people in the district of Kaifabad live in the city itself. The district includes several smaller outlying cities, as well as vast rural areas—some agricultural and settled with small villages, others mostly uninhabited.

I had agreed to meet Dr. Ibrahim, the WHO foreign consultant assigned to the district of Kaifabad, a few days before the door-to-door polio campaign began.[1] Our meeting was at his office, which the government provided for him in the district health administration building. While I had worked in Kaifabad before, this was my first time working with Dr. Ibrahim; WHO consultants were routinely switched from district to district. I arrived before he did and waited on a paint-spattered wooden bench in the hallway outside his padlocked metal door. The floors in the hallway were grimy, though the paint on the walls was fresh enough not to have peeled, the way paint seemed to do everywhere in Kaifabad. When Dr. Ibrahim arrived, he greeted me warmly, unlocked the door, and invited me into the office, which was furnished with a large desk and some cane chairs that had seen better days. He asked me to sit and got out his laptop.

The first order of business was to meet the executive director of health, the EDO, for the district of Kaifabad, the man responsible for overseeing all health activities in the district. I had met the EDO before when I had worked in Kaifabad, but Dr. Ibrahim felt that protocol demanded a formal meeting to describe my participation in this campaign. We went across the courtyard to the EDO's large, wood-paneled office, its imposing desk covered in green felt and decorated with a "stop TB" plaque. As we waited for the EDO to arrive, I asked Dr. Ibrahim about his career path. He was from northern Africa and had worked in Pakistan before. Dr. Ibrahim mentioned that most WHO employees did not covet the Kaifabad post because the city was so large and the district so political. At the time I wondered what he meant, exactly, by "political."

When the EDO arrived, we were all served tea. We made small talk in English, as Dr. Ibrahim did not speak Urdu and the EDO's English was impeccable. Dr. Ibrahim mentioned that in one area, workers had not shown up for training; the EDO said he would fire the area's supervisor. Dr. Ibrahim added that he and I were happy to be able to "support" the campaign in Kaifabad. One of the EDO's assistants, sitting to the side of the office, said that the district was grateful for our "help." The EDO looked at his watch, we all stood up, and Dr. Ibrahim and I were escorted out of the room.

Over the next two days, I attended a number of training sessions for workers responsible for administering polio vaccine. They were being trained by their "area in charge"; most of the trainings were at local health posts. Training, which all workers had to attend each round, covered how vaccine was to be administered and how houses, children, and record sheets were to be labeled to confirm vaccination. In my role as supervisor, I was supposed to verify that trainings were taking place, that all workers were in attendance, and that the information provided was complete and accurate. Dr. Ibrahim was doing similar work, as were ten government doctors, called "campaign support persons," whom WHO paid extra to work on the polio campaign.

The quality of the training varied widely. At one session, a few people drinking tea on a tiny couch in an even tinier living room claimed that just minutes before my arrival, twenty people had been in that very room, but that the training had concluded quickly and all had left. At another, the area in charge gave a clear, interactive presentation with all his workers present and participating—including extra workers the area in charge paid out of his own meager wages just in case one of the regular workers got sick or had a family emergency.

One training session I attended was at an area in charge's small two-room home, with a double bed and a small sofa in one room and a kitchen in the other. Present were about ten or twelve men, all railway employees, and a couple of women. The women were lady health workers, employees of the government's Health Department; the men were so-called volunteers, the label for anyone recruited to work on polio eradication who was not a regular employee of the Ministry of Health. Neither these men nor any volunteers I encountered in Pakistan freely offered their work without pay; they worked on polio eradication for the money (or because, as in the case of these railway workers, it was a requirement), though they were quick to note that at around two dollars a day, it was hardly worth it. The women were in the kitchen when I arrived; they came out to greet me and the men were cleared off the small couch so we women could all sit there. The men all crowded onto the bed. The area in charge gave the training in this small living room, writing on the back of an old polio poster and speaking over the whirring of a large standing fan. None of the employees were new; most had participated in many trainings, and many polio campaigns, over the years. One of the men asked, "How long will we have to keep doing this?" The area in charge responded, "As long as they keep sending money from abroad."

At all the trainings, lady health workers and other employees of the Health Department who were working on the campaign were usually present, while volunteers were often absent. One campaign support person, a young doctor, discussed this issue with me. After a training we both attended in the operating room of a health post, where all nine lady health workers were present and all five volunteers—teachers at a nearby school—were absent, the campaign support person said: "The EDO doesn't lean on the education department to get the teachers to attend trainings, or even to send volunteers at all—if one school refuses to send them, the rest of the schools say, 'Then why are we sending them?' It's really hard for this zonal supervisor to find teams—I don't know where he gets them from."[2]

As the government's Health Department did not have a large enough

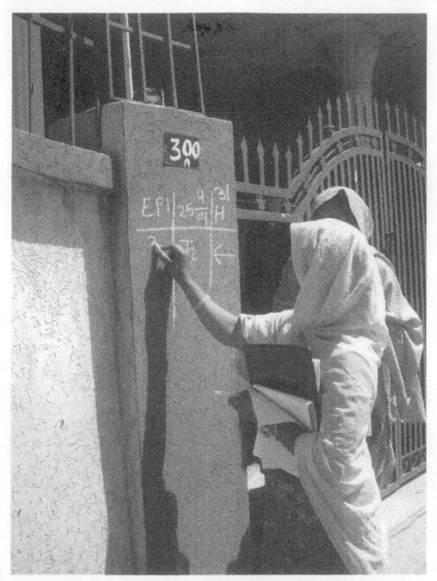

Lady health workers chalk-marking a house. They mark the date, the team number, the number of children immunized, the number of children remaining unimmunized, and the direction they are traveling. Photo by author.

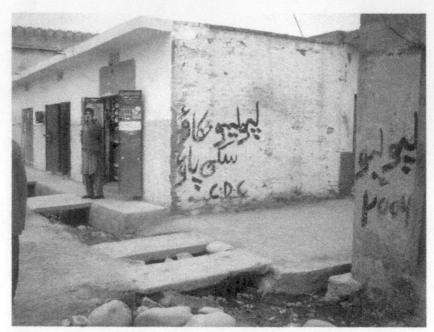

Streetscape in rural Kaifabad. An enthusiastic government official painted pro-vaccination slogans on the walls several years ago. The open sewers are typical of Kaifabad. Photo by author.

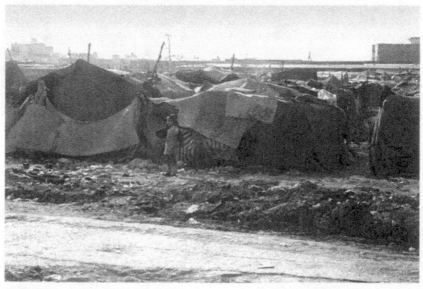

Urban slum in Kaifabad. Photo by author.

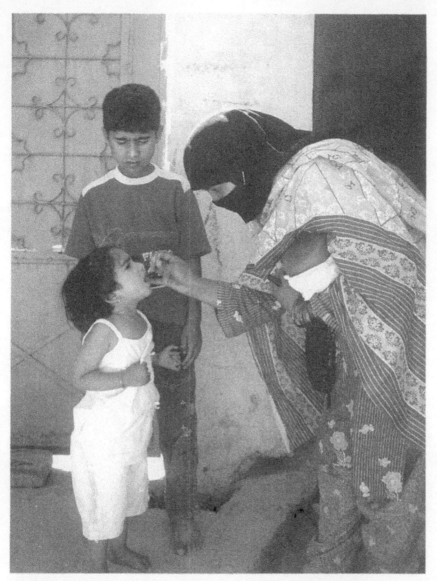

A lady health worker gives polio vaccine to a child in Kaifabad. Photo
by author.

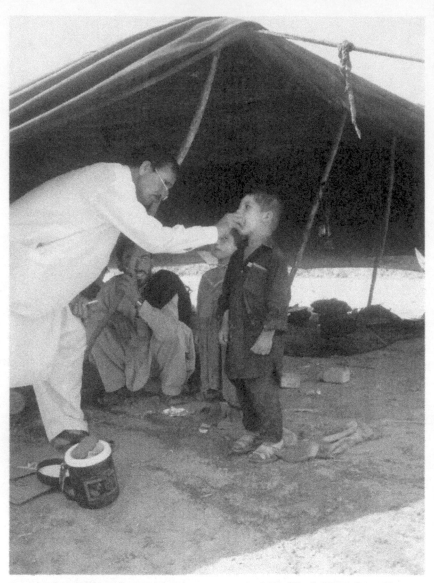

A nomadic child is vaccinated in his tent in rural Kaifabad. Note the cooler in the lower left corner of the picture; these are filled with ice and used to keep vaccine cold as teams travel door-to-door. Photo by author.

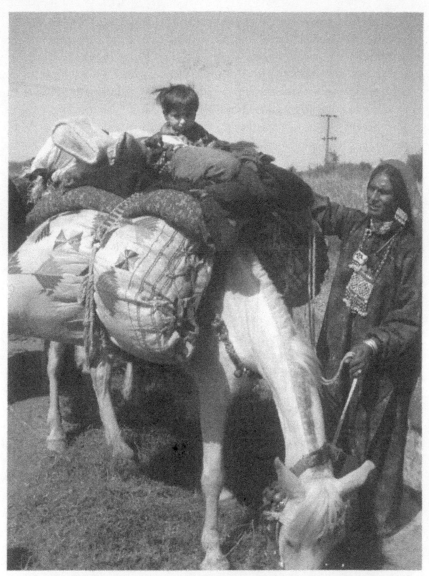

A nomadic child travels through Kaifabad district. The child was vaccinated by a team working at a transit point at a major intersection. Photo by author.

workforce to carry out the campaigns on its own—200,000 ground-level workers were needed across Pakistan—difficulties in obtaining volunteers from outside the health sector were ongoing. These were exacerbated by the low pay the volunteers, like the lady health workers working on polio eradication, received; they usually earned no pay at all for attending training.[3] The lady health workers, and other Health Department employees, could be coerced into participating in polio campaigns even for low pay under the threat of losing their regular jobs. No such threat existed for the volunteers.

Kaifabad was a tightly run district, and its lady health workers reported for duty. In other districts, lady health workers as well as volunteers skipped trainings. Tanveer's sister-in-law was a lady health worker in another district. While she worked on polio, she never attended trainings, and this round was no exception. "Why would I go to a training when they don't even give me the thirty rupees [fifty cents] they're supposed to, and it costs me over a hundred rupees to get there and back?" she asked Tanveer.

The day before the campaign begins, WHO and UNICEF insist that it be inaugurated by key government officials as part of social mobilization for the district. This time, Kaifabad's inauguration, at one of the district's hospitals, would feature the district *nazim*, the highest elected official in Kaifabad. When Tanveer and I arrived at the hospital (a little late), we were ushered into the pediatric ward through hallways packed with people waiting for medical care; there, the *nazim* gave drops to three or four children while a few photographers took pictures. Only we who were involved in the campaign and the people who happened to be in the hospital were present. Next, we were escorted to the tiled office of the hospital director, where about fifteen people, including high-level district health officials and various *chamcha*s (*ćamća*, literally, "spoons," political flunkies who make a career of flattering people in power), were served tea, meat patties, and biscuits. When the *nazim* got up to leave, we all stood and rushed after him in what Tanveer called the "*chamcha* parade." The *nazim* got into his white Corolla and drove off, and the inauguration was over.

# The Campaign

## *Day 1*

On the first day of the campaign, I was assigned to monitor work in Amirkhan, a rural area outside the city. Tanveer and I drove there on the Grand Trunk Road, the chaotic highway choked with heavily decorated trucks that crosses the northern Punjab from Lahore to Peshawar. Our first stop was along the highway at a transit point set up to vaccinate children waiting to board buses and vans. Other teams were going door-to-door at the same time; vaccinating children at the transit point was one of several methods employed to reach children who might not be at home when the team visited. Two teams of three men each worked at this transit point, one on each side of the road. They all wore yellow bibs identifying them as polio workers and were doing excellent work. One man rounded up children from families headed toward the buses, while the other two vaccinated them under the shade of an army-green tent (the vaccine is heat sensitive, and in the summer must be kept out of the sun).[4] The team members procured chairs from somewhere for Tanveer and me and placed them under the tent; they tried to purchase sodas for us, but we resisted, saying truthfully that we had just drunk some in the car on the way over. Many of the children being vaccinated in this tent were traveling with their grandfathers, who told them to open their mouths to get the drops of vaccine and Vitamin A. One little girl whose clothing identified her as Pathan, perhaps from Afghanistan, had bleeding sores all around her mouth. She was, of necessity, vaccinated and sent on; the team members at the transit posts did not have the time, the materials, or the training to treat her.

The teams had called the zonal supervisor, a level above the area in charge, on his cell phone when we got to Amirkhan, and he soon arrived to meet us. He got into the back seat of my tiny Toyota, and Tanveer turned off the Grand Trunk Road onto nearly empty rural asphalt roads that led to nearby villages. It was harvest time for wheat, and everywhere people were in the fields working—men, women, children, and the old. It was hot, and the neatly tied bundles of wheat propped in circular formations glinted in the bright sunlight. That this campaign happened to fall during the harvest made things difficult for team members on two counts: their own families needed them for harvest work, and they had to track down children playing in the fields as their parents worked.

We stopped at a basic health unit, the village primary health center, painted the standard dark red; I checked to make sure that routine vaccination was going on as usual inside. Then we attempted to find the nearest team going house-to-house. This proved a challenge. We walked around, and then drove around, for over an hour; we found where the team had been and where they had not yet been, but we could find no sign of them. The driving was very slow going over the rutted earth road; once we had to stop because a cow had stretched its rope tether across the road like a roadblock. The team might have stopped for lunch somewhere, and there was no way for us to know where. I was mildly annoyed by the wild goose chase, though I did my best not to show it; the area in charge, who was supposed to know where his teams were, was frantic and defensive.

Finally we gave up and looked for another team, which we found right away—two plump women chalking on houses near the paved road. I looked at their tally sheet, where they had recorded the number of children vaccinated in various age groups; I counted their empty and full vials of vaccine. As all supervisors are taught to do, to screen for imprecise or falsified tallying, I did a quick calculation in my head to make sure the number of children reported vaccinated was consistent with the amount of vaccine used. I checked to make sure that they were recording children not at home when they visited a given residence, and that these children added up to at least 5 percent of the total children immunized. I knocked on the doors of a few nearby homes to verify that the team had chalked the correct numbers on the door, detailing the number of children under five living in the house and the number vaccinated that day. By this, my fourth time working on a polio campaign, I had gotten pretty good at assessing the quality of work a team was doing. This team's work was meticulous and thorough. I told them that it looked excellent, and the lady health worker beamed.

"It's a joy to be checked," she said, "because then someone sees and appreciates my work."

The work of the other teams we checked that day was good too. In rural areas of Kaifabad like this one, there were enough lady health workers for nearly every team to have one, and teams knew the families whose homes they were visiting.

In the evening, all the supervisors met in the office of Amirkhan's highest health official, gathering on chairs around the official's large glass-topped desk crowned with several penholders. As usual in these meetings, of the fifteen or so people present, I was the only woman and the only foreigner. I also seemed to be the person with the most power. When sodas

arrived in glass bottles, I was served first. When the official called Dr. Ibrahim on the phone to update him on the day's work and Dr. Ibrahim asked
to speak to me, someone jumped up to carry the phone and cord around
the room to me so that I would not have to move. (Dr. Ibrahim told me
that the work he had seen that day in the city of Kaifabad was "very bad.")
When the meeting, which was fairly low-key as there did not seem to have
been any major problems, seemed to be over, everyone waited for me to
make a move before they got up from their chairs.

## Day 2

At a basic health unit in the outskirts of the city, I said hello to the doctor, a youngish woman whom I had met during training. She wore heavy
eyeliner, sprayed the top of her hair into a puff, and was getting a master
of public health degree via distance learning from the London School of
Hygiene. A plaque on her desk read "Best Doctor of 2003, Kaifabad."

The doctor called the area in charge for this area to meet us, a lady
health supervisor in the lady health worker program. When she finally
arrived, she said she had taken a taxi to the basic health unit—women in
Pakistan cannot ride on motorbikes, the transport provided for area in
charges. The taxi fare was half her daily wage.

We visited four teams, hers and those of another area in charge. As
we walked around this newly urbanizing area under the hot sun, the lady
health supervisor apologized for the smell from the open gutters. Most of
the work was good, although one team had done its work the night before,
when it was cooler, but had chalked today's date on the doors.

We were called back to the basic health unit to greet Dr. Hyder, a
government doctor hired by WHO as a campaign support person on this
campaign. I knew Dr. Hyder fairly well from previous work in the district.
When Dr. Hyder arrived, he, the doctor, the lady health supervisor, and I
drank tea in the doctor's office, leaving the doctor's hapless patients to wait
in line in the dusty entranceway to the unit. As the conversation turned to
health unit politics, the doctor brusquely directed the lady health supervisor to leave the room, and she did.

Dr. Hyder then asked me to spend several hours checking work with
him. I resisted; I felt it was a waste of resources to have two supervisors
traveling together. But Dr. Hyder played his trump card. "You're here to
support us," he said. And so I followed him to several areas and then did
more work on my own with Tanveer later in the afternoon.

The evening meetings in the city of Kaifabad proper were very different from those in outlying Amirkhan. These were large meetings of more than fifty people, with everyone from the area in charges on up in attendance and expected to speak briefly about any problems encountered during the day. The meeting room was large, with lots of aging chairs upholstered in brown cloth, peeling white paint on the walls, and slowly revolving ceiling fans. While I often tried to avoid a position of prominence, always being the only woman, this time I ended up sitting in front next to the podium and microphone with the EDO, Dr. Ibrahim, and other high-ranking officials, facing everyone else.

Before the meeting started, I discussed how the campaign was going with Dr. Ahmed, a Pakistani WHO employee assigned to Kaifabad, who was sitting next to me. I said things seemed to be fine and mentioned the team that had done the work last night but seemed to have done a good job. Dr. Ahmed shrugged and smiled wryly. "Sometimes we have to ignore such things," he said. This was a very different reaction from that of Dr. Ibrahim, who had been quite upset about the situation when I had spoken to him on the phone that morning.

That was not all Dr. Ibrahim had been upset about. He had expressed to me, and to others, his concern that workers were not getting an early enough start. Dr. Ibrahim, as always extraordinarily hardworking, had gone to an outlying area of Kaifabad in the afternoon and had not made it back by the time the meeting began. The meeting opened with widespread dissatisfaction with the absent Dr. Ibrahim.

One zonal supervisor stood up and stated that at one basic health unit Dr. Ibrahim visited, seven out of twelve teams had collected their supplies and were out working by 8:30 in the morning. Apparently Dr. Ibrahim was dissatisfied that *all* teams had not yet arrived. "How early are they supposed to leave?" the supervisor asked angrily. Dr. Ibrahim had also objected to an area in charge's keeping vaccine in the freezer at his home. But, the zonal supervisor said he had cleared out all the food, and there was no other freezer available nearby.

The EDO and Dr. Ahmed addressed these and similar complaints. The EDO did not deny their validity, but said that people need to "compromise" with Dr. Ibrahim. Dr. Ahmed suggested using a government freezer at a nearby railway station.

"The foreigners who come to check are out to get us," someone said.

"That's not true. Madam here," said the EDO, indicating me, "said the work in Amirkhan was excellent."

In the structure of district meetings in Kaifabad, the lowest-ranking people spoke first. I spoke third to last, before only Dr. Ibrahim (who came in the middle of the meeting) and the EDO. When it was Dr. Ahmed's turn, he was asked to speak in English so that Dr. Ibrahim could understand—the comprehension of the probably forty or so people present who did not speak English being, apparently, secondary.

While Dr. Ahmed was speaking, the EDO interrupted to severely scold a worker who Dr. Ahmed said was "harsh" with female workers, then followed up by saying, in Urdu, that he would fire people who weren't doing their jobs. "We terminated three people," he said, "and I heard about it from my wife before she would even give me my breakfast." Apparently the wife of one of the people who had been fired had come to the EDO's wife in tears. The EDO said he was unmoved. "We need people who are going to work. If people need money, then they should work."

Dr. Ahmed then continued with his talk. He mentioned Dr. Ibrahim's concerns about a block of ice for keeping vaccine cold that was delivered before the basic health unit opened and placed over an open sewer. Dr. Ibrahim had been worried about possible contamination.

The area in charge in question stood up. "Sir, it was propped outside the door."

The EDO cut him off, in English. "What the hell you are doing, yār?"

When it was Dr. Ibrahim's turn to speak, he stood behind the podium to give a long introductory talk, ending with the conclusion of the day: "Sad to say it was not a good outcome." The problems he mentioned were largely the ones discussed before his arrival: he said that teams were not starting early enough and argued that vaccine should be in temperature-controlled storage rather than a house fridge where the electricity could go out, "or there could be any other mishap."

Dr. Ibrahim talked for a long time. When he was finished, the EDO said: "We have a shortage of human resource within the city, you must acknowledge. We are managing with volunteers; . . . we are under the great pressure."

"The second thing," the EDO continued, "is that you visited one health institution at seven a.m.," when realistic times to monitor are 8:30 a.m. to 4 p.m. "There should be some compromise. I appreciate your activity, but—"

"Okay," Dr. Ibrahim smiled. "That's true."

A high-level government official then stood at the podium and addressed the assembled in Urdu. "Dr. Ibrahim didn't say you couldn't keep vaccine in your homes," he said. "He just said you had to have a thermometer and ice packs in case the electricity goes out. This seems to be a communications problem—complaints have gotten blown out of proportion."

This was certainly true, I thought, and probably due to the language barrier between Dr. Ibrahim and most area in charges.

The official concluded the meeting with an exhortation to work hard. "Each of you should think, if—God forbid—a polio case occurs in my area, then who will be responsible?"

## *Day 3*

Tanveer and I started the day with Dr. Hyder, who had asked my assistance in dealing with the headmaster of a refusal school, a man we had both met before. During a campaign several months previously, the area in charge of that area had reported that a school with a large number of under-five children was refusing to let vaccinators enter. Dr. Hyder and I had gone then to speak with the headmaster of the school.

The school was in an aging townhouse development on the outskirts of the city, a place perhaps not for the very rich, but at least for the upwardly mobile. The school's courtyard was a large spotless expanse with expensive playground equipment and a view over the rows of cement townhomes. On our first visit, during the previous campaign, Dr. Hyder and I went to the headmaster's office and were told he was with some parents; could we wait a few minutes? We watched the clock as these few minutes stretched into half an hour, then forty-five minutes, then an hour. Nearly an hour and a half passed and Dr. Hyder and I were beginning to get irate when we were finally ushered into the office of the headmaster. Our anger stemmed from the fact that campaign days were busy ones and we had a lot of other work to do, but probably also from the fact that within the Health Department during campaign days, we were the most important people everywhere we went; everyone *else* had to wait for *us*.

The headmaster, ex-military, was a silver-haired gentleman in a suit who apologized fairly insincerely for keeping us waiting as he met with parent after parent. Dr. Hyder told him who we were and why we were there.

"This is a school for the rich," the headmaster explained. "These parents, unlike others in Pakistan, are so worried about the health of their children that they make sure they get all the routine immunizations, so there is no need at all to do polio campaigns in the school." My response that immunity against polio in Pakistan required far more than the three doses of vaccine given during routine immunizations fell on deaf ears.

The headmaster started to get angry. We should not be focusing on rich schools, he insisted—we were only visiting him to "fulfill a percentage"—as these children couldn't possibly get polio. He argued that we should be focusing on the poor, who had no education, TV, or radio: "they are like cattle." Exasperated, Dr. Hyder and I said that we would have *liked* to focus on the poor, but that the headmaster had forced us to spend the whole morning with *him*. He finally agreed to let our teams vaccinate in the school, "only because you sent such a high-powered team, but I am not convinced." We left feeling stressed out and not at all victorious.

So in this campaign, several months later, the school was again a refusal, and again Dr. Hyder asked me to speak to the headmaster, this time by myself—it was clear Dr. Hyder was reluctant to go.[5] I had been dreading the encounter with the headmaster all night, so I told Tanveer I wanted to get it done with as soon as possible in the morning. Tanveer, who had waited in the car the last time we had gone in, said he wanted to come with me and see the headmaster for himself.

Tanveer and I met the area in charge and the team members by the school, and we headed in. Trying a new technique, I told the secretary that I was very pressed for time. I can't wait, I said, because I have work in the field, but if the headmaster wants to give me a time I will show up at that time to meet with him. No, no, the secretary said, the headmaster is here and he will not make you wait. I sat down. After thirty seconds I told the secretary again, really, I'm not prepared to wait. The secretary discreetly called the headmaster in his office and then told me to go ahead and vaccinate the children. This was wonderful news. It was a great relief not to have to argue with the headmaster, and the area in charge and the teams were happy too, and got to work immediately. We left in a congratulatory mood.

Driving along the road away from the school, I saw clothes drying on a temporary hut in a ravine near a wide dirty river. Tanveer drove over the bridge and parked, and we walked down past a bus stand, past an area where buffaloes were tethered in makeshift stables, to the small hut where a woman sat nursing one infant while another small boy played on the dirt floor. There were a lot of flies. She said no, no team had come to vaccinate her children. I wasn't surprised, because you wouldn't know this house existed from where the teams were working in established neighborhoods. We called the area in charge to tell him. He thanked us and said he would let the team know.

Previous research I had done on vaccination coverage in Kaifabad had shown that nomads, beggars, and other people living in temporary housing were much less likely to receive vaccine than the general population—coverage rates in those populations were less than 80 percent, far below the target of 95 percent.[6] I had been assigned to Kaifabad on this campaign with the hope that I would focus on these populations, and that this attention would lead to improved coverage.

So we moved on to another area where Dr. Hyder had told us there was a tent colony. The area in charge met us nearby and led the way there on his motorcycle. By this time, it was late morning and punishingly hot. Tanveer parked in front of a store by a large and busy street. We scrambled up a dirty hill beside the street and crossed the road on a railroad trestle, stepping from tie to tie; thankfully there was a metal floor of sorts a couple of feet beneath the tracks. The settlement of ragged tents, invisible from the road, was here. The team had visited the area and gone to each tent, but asking around, we found four children who had gone unvaccinated because they were out begging with their parents when the team came.

One of them was a four-month-old with diarrhea. Her grandmother held her on a *chār-pāī* (a wood-and-rope bed), partially shaded by a tent pieced together from pieces of dirty fabric. The city trash had been beaten back, but it threatened to take over the home. Flies were everywhere. The parents asked me what to do about the child's diarrhea, and for once I knew what to say.[7] We found a few other missed children a little apart from the main settlement, playing near a large and polluted river under the shade of the railroad bridge.

In the evening, Tanveer and I saw another tent population from the road, not in Kaifabad but in the neighboring district, which was less well managed. By now, the evening of the third day of the campaign, the teams were supposed to have visited every house in Pakistan once. Days four and five of the campaign are supposed to be devoted to revisiting houses where children were not at home on the first pass.

These tent colonies, though, had not been visited. Tanveer and I vaccinated twenty or twenty-five children under five, some in open tents in the sun, others in half-mud, half-tent structures, and a few in more permanent homes. Most of the children had scabies, an itchy rash caused by mites, and many had infected sores from scratching their bodies. One child of about a year and a half, my son's age, had recently been horribly burned when she fell into a clay oven; she was lying in a metal cradle. Her legs were in bandages, but her injuries were so severe that her feet were facing backward. The mother asked me what she should do, and I was useless. Ask a doctor, I said. Such are the moments when I think I should have gone to medical school.

Inside another house we found two children. The house was one very large, very dark cement room; it took me a few moments to see the two children, one sitting on the floor amid masses of flies, and one sleeping on a bed. The boy on the floor had diarrhea, the mother told me, and I said it was okay to vaccinate him nonetheless. We woke up the baby girl on the bed to vaccinate her. Because there was so little light, I didn't realize right away that the child's diarrhea was all over the floor (they couldn't have afforded diapers)—which explained the flies. I got diarrhea on the edges of my *dupaṭṭā*, the large cotton shawl I wore over my head. When we left, I asked the neighbor's daughter for water, which she brought in a jug from a large clay pot, and I rinsed my shawl.

Everyone we came across in this area was extremely friendly and helpful. They urged us to stay for tea, to have some food, but we had to get back to Kaifabad for the evening meeting. On the way back into the city, securely jammed in traffic in the gathering dusk, Tanveer and I both called the houses we were staying in. Both had gone unvisited by the teams, our children thus far uncovered.

## Day 4

In the morning, my friend Shama and I took my son for a walk around the neighborhood where we were living to see how many houses had been missed. We walked up and down the streets just wide enough for a subcompact car, with open gutters and a fog of flies. There was no chalking anywhere, and when we yelled out to some of our neighbors, they told us nobody had come for polio. The entire sector of about a hundred houses had been missed, including two schools. We came across a polio team of two women a few streets over. I was carrying my son, and when I asked the team about the coverage of this area, they were impatient with me— clearly they thought I was some random woman who was upset that her child had not been covered. "That's not our area," they said. As I didn't have a copy of the maps for this area showing which team was responsible for which streets, I didn't know whether they were telling the truth.[8] When I explained who I was—accustomed now to being seen as a person of importance—they said they would give my phone number to their area in charge when he came by.

Shama asked me how much these women were paid. I told her about two dollars a day. "Well," Shama observed, "obviously you're not going to get good work out of somebody for that much. I could sit at home sewing and earn twice that, and I wouldn't have to be out in the sun."

The area in charge found Shama and me talking to a friend in front of the tiny corner store with its inventory of dusty biscuit packages and Pepsi. He apologized for the area not being covered and blamed it on the team I met, which he said was new and unsure about which areas were its responsibility; the story the zonal supervisor had given me on the phone was that one of the team member's mothers had suddenly become deathly ill.

Shortly after this, I left with Tanveer to work elsewhere. In the evening, Shama told me there was a great commotion when the contingent of supervisors came to the door, all of them—the zonal supervisor, the area in charge, the team—asking Shama where I had gone and whom I had told about this area, my son crying, the boy from upstairs yelling, then the supervisors telling Shama that the whole area is now covered, the schools are covered, tell madam not to worry.

Tanveer got a phone call from the zonal supervisor as we were checking some tent colonies that had been poorly covered in the last campaign. Within minutes, the area in charge, Fahad, showed up with a team of two young men on his motorcycle. Obviously, word of my whereabouts had gotten around. There were still a lot of missed children, but Fahad assured me he would cover them in the evening with his son.

## Day 5

In the morning Tanveer and I went to Malakot, another small city on the outskirts of the district. Driving in, we came across a large group of Bakarwals, nomadic goat herders, with hundreds of goats and a long train of horses. The children with them, wrapped in colorful blankets and secured atop bell-bedecked horses, had been vaccinated by the teams working at major road intersections. We had a long discussion about whether three other young children ahead in the camp (hidden somewhere in the hills) had been covered; the men had their doubts, but their mother said they had been vaccinated, and mothers are usually the ones to believe. However, the mother also remarked that she couldn't believe that some people (us) had nothing better to do than follow other people (them) around for no reason. As we stood talking to them, a busload of Japanese tourists pulled over to the side of the road to take pictures.

Next, we stopped at a settlement of beggars beside the railroad tracks. The area in charge who was with us had rechecked the entire settlement that morning, and we could not find a single missed child. The settlement was filthy; the people very polite. They thanked us for coming—"May Allah keep you happy."

Driving along the road, we saw some other tents in the distance. Tanveer turned off the paved road and drove over the hard clay toward them. The tents were in a large and beautiful grove of tall thin trees, shady in the hot day. In the first clean large tent we approached, made of a sheet of gray canvas stretched more or less horizontally over somewhat dusty handmade blankets, we found six children under five, all unvaccinated; they had come this morning from a neighboring district, and before that from Amirkhan. From this tent we could see another through the trees (five uncovered children), and from that another (seven more uncovered children), and from that another (six more), and from that some more (all covered, having come from Kaifabad). We vaccinated the children and marked the tents with chalk. The work was pleasant, the area beautiful; the children played in a stream that ran through the grove. To find so many missed children in one place was worrisome. The zonal supervisor with us assured us repeatedly that he undoubtedly would have found and covered these children this morning; he also pointed out several times that since these children had just arrived this morning, no workers in Malakot had been negligent. He was right, but this was part of the reason nomads so often slipped through the cracks, and why nomadic populations sometimes sustain polio's circulation.

We went back to Kaifabad for a meeting in the afternoon. Dr. Ibrahim headed the meeting; Dr. Ahmed, all the campaign support persons including Dr. Hyder, and I were there. The goal of the meeting was to decide who would be checking which areas during postcampaign monitoring.

During the meeting, Dr. Ibrahim said he was very dissatisfied with the campaign thus far. When I mentioned that I thought work in one area of Amirkhan was good, Dr. Ibrahim said he found a huge population of nomads there with more than 150 children that was completely uncovered. The campaign support persons said to me quietly that the area was due to be covered that night; Dr. Ibrahim was making, they thought, a big deal out of nothing. When Dr. Ibrahim left the room, a few of them discussed what they felt was his overreaction to minor issues.

Dr. Ahmed attempted damage control. "You have to understand," he said, "that if there's a case, people will blame him for it. So that's why he reacts the way he does to problems."

One campaign support person was late to the meeting because he was at the police station; one of the teams had, he said, been "beaten up" and their cell phone smashed by a family angry at the repeated visiting of their house to recheck. Dr. Ibrahim asked the campaign support person, "Were you really working or were you at home?"

The campaign support person was annoyed. "I was at home sleeping," he shot back. "Of course I was working!" He shook his head and shot an exasperated look at the other campaign support persons.

Dr. Ibrahim asked how many Union Councils (an administrative division) one person could reasonably check during postcampaign monitoring. In the previous round, we had each monitored four per day. I said that I thought that while one person could check four Union Councils per day in the city of Kaifabad, three was a more reasonable number in rural areas, where driving long distances was necessary. This sentiment was widely echoed by the campaign support persons, and Dr. Ibrahim agreed that quality was more important than quantity. On the wings of this success, Dr. Hyder tried unsuccessfully to get Dr. Ibrahim to lower the workload further by giving his permission to take off a national holiday that fell during the monitoring days.

Dr. Ibrahim decided in the course of the meeting to bring in four additional monitors from neighboring provinces because, he said, he was concerned about campaign quality in so many areas. No opposition was voiced to this idea. I knew Dr. Ibrahim wanted monitors from outside the district because he did not trust the campaign support persons, who were government employees most of the time, to remain immune from pressure to falsify data. That they did, in fact, falsify data was almost without question; I had seen results from the previous round, where several had claimed to have checked more than six hundred children and not found a single one unvaccinated. As the odd child was always missed even in the very best areas, such results were impossible. Dr. Ibrahim hoped that monitors from other districts could resist political pressure and deliver more accurate results.

For this reason, Dr. Ibrahim assigned the areas where he was most concerned about the quality of work to the monitors he trusted: himself, Dr. Ahmed, and me. The negotiation of who would check where was extraordinarily inefficient, and the meeting dragged on for three hours. Afterward, there was a meeting of the rest of the staff, including area in charges, zonal supervisors, and the EDO. I opted not to attend: it was already 5:30, I knew I had three very long days ahead, and my young son got upset when I was not home on time in the evenings. If I'd known how interesting the meeting would prove to be, I would have attended it anyway.

## Postcampaign Monitoring

### Day 1

In the morning, Tanveer and I drove to the area of the city where our assigned Union Councils were located. We called the area in charge of the first Union Council, who was supposed to meet us and show us around the area. He was surprised that we had come that day and protested that we weren't supposed to be there. Tanveer maneuvered our car into a tiny spot between an ice-cream machine and a school van, half on the grimy sidewalk littered with plastic bags, and half on the street clogged with cars, bicycles, motorcycle rickshaws, and school children. The stores on the street were opening, rolling up their metal shutters, and while we waited, Tanveer and I sat in the car and drank tea out of chipped china cups from a nearby vendor.

When the area in charge arrived half an hour later, he said that teams were still working in two of the Union Councils I was supposed to check that day and that I should check them some other day. I was annoyed that teams were still working three days after they were to have covered all their areas. I said truthfully that I didn't have free time on other days to come back and check these two Union Councils, a good four or five hours of work. The area in charge left for a moment and returned with a phone call for me on his cell phone from a high-level government official. The official told me that on the order of the EDO, I was not allowed to check in this area of Kaifabad today.

I was surprised, as I had never heard of monitors not being permitted to do their jobs. I called Dr. Ibrahim, who said that the moratorium on monitoring certain areas had been decided at last night's meeting, but by the time the meeting concluded it had been late, he had been upset, and he had forgotten to call and tell me. After our meeting in the afternoon, several campaign support persons had told the EDO that Dr. Ibrahim was bringing in external monitors without the EDO's permission. They apparently framed this as Dr. Ibrahim sneaking around under the EDO's nose. Dr. Ibrahim said that yesterday he had been trying to contact the EDO all day regarding additional external monitors, but that the EDO was unavailable in a meeting, and then not answering his phone. Dr. Ibrahim said that Dr. Ahmed supported his version of events.

At the evening meeting, apparently, the EDO was upset and other high-level officials were angry, categorically refusing to accept any external monitors. This was, from my perspective, a surprising development. At a recent meeting in Islamabad with representatives from Geneva present, government and WHO officials had stressed that external monitors were a very important aspect of good campaigns. The problem discussed at the Islamabad meeting had been the procurement of such monitors, certainly not the acceptance of them.

Dr. Ibrahim told me on the phone that, at the meeting the night before, he had outlined the reasons for requesting external monitors. He was concerned about the quality of the campaign: he had seen many substandard areas during his work over a few days, and he had seen only a small fraction of the total area of the district. As the existing monitors could monitor only about half of Kaifabad's Union Councils, he wanted to bring in external monitors to evaluate more areas. This would presumably turn up more areas that had been poorly covered and thus could be re-covered. He had capped this by saying he was very concerned that with the current campaign quality, there could be a polio case in the district, which would be disastrous for the EDO.

The EDO, who was trying to broker a compromise, had responded that two of the four external monitors would be allowed to work but that he should be the one to choose the external monitors. This was not acceptable to Dr. Ibrahim, who said he would bring this issue to the attention of provincial officials.

Thus last night's meeting had ended in an impasse. Since then, Dr. Ibrahim had told WHO and government officials at the provincial level about this, and he reported that they were "very upset" and that they found such behavior "unacceptable." They told Dr. Ibrahim that if the district administrators were going to make such unreasonable requests, they had to put them in writing so the province could address the issue. However, the EDO was evading putting his decision in writing, saying he would do it later. Dr. Ibrahim wrote his own letter describing the situation, which I later read. It described the bare facts without any breath of suggestion that there was a conflict.

At any rate, one fallout of the whole debacle was the EDO's statement that, since it appeared there were so many problems in parts of the city, he would give workers in those areas an extra day to work on their vaccination before postcampaign monitoring began. Thus I had been asked to leave the area I had been assigned to. I should, I was told, check a different area instead.

Dr. Ibrahim then asked me if I knew anyone who could go with him as an interpreter when he checked areas that day—someone from outside the polio program. He just needed, he said, someone to tell him what answers parents were giving to his questions; otherwise even if children were unvaccinated, the area in charges present could cover it up. Dr. Ibrahim planned to pay the person something reasonable out of his own pocket (which given his extraordinarily high salary was not a hardship). I suggested someone, we set up a meeting, and we all set off.

Before we even got to the area we were supposed to check, we got a phone call from the area in charge, Fahad. I'd met him before, and I liked him.

"Are you really coming today?" he asked. "We're not ready—most of the area in charges are not here."

I told him he could just show me his area first. Later, I learned that all the workers from Fahad's area had been dispatched to cover other areas of the city.

We began with a tent colony that had been poorly covered the other day, a large beggar's colony in a dusty clearing between homes under construction and next to a mountain of garbage. Fahad had, as he told me he would, done vaccinations in the evening with his son, and I was not able to find an uncovered child. The problem came later, in a street of middle-class homes; we stopped at a house chalked "0," for no children, but I saw children upstairs and called up. A woman came to the balcony. She had three young children, all uncovered. We vaccinated them; evidently she was not there when the team came. Because there were three children, the area qualified as a "red area," and I would write up a report.

As we walked away from the area, Fahad said, "Can you do something? Just make those children fewer than three, because I'm going to get into a lot of trouble with the EDO."

"I can't," I said.

"If you hadn't done checking today, and I'd had an extra day," Fahad said, "I would have covered those children."

A little later, we came across a house chalked R for refusal and inhabited by an undoubtedly strange man who said that his child had not been immunized but then disappeared inside the house, not to return. As we were standing in front of the house, fruitlessly calling through the doorway, the man's ten-year-old daughter passed us on her way in. Tanveer asked her to bring her young sibling out to be immunized, and she did. Her father always acted like this, she said. And I marked another missed child in Fahad's area.

As we got back into the car, Fahad said: "Please do something about all these missed children. I have three young children; we rent our flat. I can't afford to have my pay stopped for months, and it will be devastating for my family if I am fired. The EDO said that this time, anyone with more than two missed children in monitoring could expect to lose their jobs."

When Fahad left, the zonal supervisor started in. "Fahad is a great worker; I'd hate to lose him."

## Day 2

In the morning, Tanveer and I set out for Sabazkot, a mountainous area outside the city. On the road there I got a phone call from Dr. Ibrahim, who asked where I had worked the day before. I replied that I had worked where he had directed me to, not where I had originally been assigned, which satisfied him.

He later explained that the EDO had received five letters of complaint about me, stating that I was conducting monitoring in parts of the city against the EDO's orders. The EDO referred these letters to another official, who called in Dr. Ibrahim and Dr. Ahmed. After they called me, they told the official that while I had gone to the area where monitoring was banned, I had been called back before beginning and had done no work there. Both Dr. Ibrahim and Dr. Ahmed had apologized to the official for forgetting to call and inform me of the monitoring ban before I drove out there.

Dr. Ibrahim told me later that I shouldn't worry about this incident, as the official was "laughing" about it. Dr. Ibrahim said he tried to press the official to take action against the people who had written the letters with false information. However, Dr. Ibrahim said, the official didn't seem concerned and just put the letters aside.

When Tanveer and I arrived at the health offices in Sabazkot, no one was there but the night guard and a peon (the official title of the lowest-level employees), both very friendly. We tried to call one of the area in charges, Javaria, a lady health supervisor, but her phone was off. The zonal supervisor was also unreachable. In the health office, there were no plans showing who was to vaccinate which area and no vaccines. The peon insisted that he knew the area and that we could get vaccines and plans at the hospital, so we took him with us. At the hospital polio vaccination post, there were no vaccines and no plans. Finally, having procured vaccine and a cooler from another part of the hospital, we chipped some ice off the side of a freezer and set off.

The peon, who was also a team member, insisted that we check his area. As I expected based on his insistence, I didn't find a missed child.

But there was a problem with recording the data, because he didn't know what Union Council he worked in. Or where the other teams' areas were, or what Union Councils they worked in. As we had no written plans, doing further monitoring was proving difficult. But we moved down the mountain on the steep and zigzagging city streets and found chalking that indicated another team's area. We found a missed child there. Shortly after that, Javaria and the zonal supervisor appeared. They were incredulous that a missed child could exist in this area. They interrogated the mother themselves, and evidently she told them the same thing she told me. Javaria mumbled something to the effect that the mother must be confused about her dates.

I checked a few other areas in the villages below Sabazkot, all of which were basically fine, and then I moved on to the huge vacation houses of the rich, below the town. We came across one family who didn't come to the imposing gate of their grand second home when we rang the doorbell, although we could see the father speaking on his cell phone on the balcony. After a long period of ignoring us, he finally responded to our repeated questions: they had arrived from Kaifabad the day before, and his child had not been immunized. I asked him to bring the child down to be immunized and he went inside, but nobody reappeared. Ringing the doorbell was fruitless.

As we stood outside hoping for someone to come out, the zonal supervisor aggressively tried to convince me that I should not record this child as missed, since the family was from the city of Kaifabad and was not in Sabazkot during the campaign. He ignored my explanation that this was a national program and that national coverage rates mattered, and became louder and louder and more and more insistent.

Ultimately an older sibling of the child came out of the house and said that the child had been vaccinated by a private doctor during the last few days. As soon as the zonal supervisor heard this, he started hounding me: "Did you write it down? Write down that the child is covered!"

Pushed over the edge, I snapped back angrily: "When the child was not immunized, you said it shouldn't count against you, and now that she's immunized, you tell me to write it down?" I didn't believe the sibling's explanation; it was a favorite excuse of the elite to prevent placing their children in what they saw as our questionable and lower-class hands, a way to refuse without being seen as refusing. However, since my instructions were to determine coverage by parental history, I accepted the child as covered.[9]

The day passed more or less in this manner, though I found almost no missed children. Several times I requested to be taken to a given area only to find myself taken somewhere else. At one point, I accompanied a team member to a home quite far below the road, down a steep mountain path.

"Have the children in your house been immunized?" the team member asked an old man lying on a wooden bed in the sun. The man had difficulty responding. "God knows," he replied wearily.

The team member, who thought I wouldn't be able to understand the man, reported to me crisply: "There are two children in the house, and they've been immunized."

Again I was pushed to snap: "You got all that out of 'God knows'"?

The team member showed no signs of embarrassment. "Well," he said, "I immunized them myself."

"If I had wanted to ask *you*," I shot back, "I wouldn't have bothered climbing halfway down this mountain."

But the work was, in fact, good; we found only one missed child in two Union Councils. In the late afternoon, we moved on to our third Union Council of the day, a cluster of villages below the town of Sabazkot. The houses were spaced far apart in mountainous terrain; checking took a long time. In the first area we checked, we found a missed child, the daughter of an army major.

Although they were supposed to, no one with us was carrying any vaccine; we had given our jerry-rigged vaccine carrier to the zonal supervisor, who was in another vehicle and had not yet appeared. We asked a team member to wait for the zonal supervisor and then vaccinate the major's daughter, while we went on ahead to do additional checking. It was getting late.

Tanveer, the area in charge, and I drove to the next village. Before we reached it, we had to stop the car, as the paved road had become too narrow even for my tiny subcompact. We walked in the beautiful warm spring evening through a green mountain village blanketed with tiny white flowers. Everyone asked us to stop for tea. The area in charge knew them all, how many children they had, their names. He was soft spoken, and I liked him. We found no missed children and headed back to meet the zonal supervisor.

We saw the zonal supervisor and the peon as we were driving back, and I got out while Tanveer went to the house of the original missed child to make sure she had been covered. I asked the zonal supervisor if he had covered the child. "Oh, yes," he said.

Tanveer came back. "I just talked to the major," he almost yelled. "He's been waiting for the past hour and nobody has come! Don't lie to us!"

Being caught out did not affect the zonal supervisor's composure in the least. "Well, we'll go and vaccinate her right now," he said.

"No," Tanveer said, "we don't trust you anymore, so give us the vaccine and we'll do it ourselves."

"Oh, well, actually, we don't have any vaccine," the zonal supervisor replied. "We left it up in Sabazkot. We'll do it tomorrow."

This was not satisfactory. The zonal supervisor called the lady health worker who lived in the area and told her to go vaccinate the child "right now," but I was not at all confident that *she* had any vaccine. However, it was much too late to go back to Sabazkot and get vaccine, and we had more areas to check before night fell. As we finished our work, in another beautiful mountain village in the gathering dark, the area in charge tried to convince me that since he had visited the house of the missed child three times (a claim for which there was no corroborating evidence in the chalking), I should not record the child as missed.

On the way back to Kaifabad in the dark, the peon we picked up in the morning (who was still with us) and the afternoon's area in charge insisted that we stop for tea and spicy fried *pakoras* at the roadside stop in their village. Tanveer and I tried to resist—I was eager to get back to my son—but it was fruitless. Over the *pakoras*, the peon mentioned that Dr. Ibrahim had finished checking in his area and had found him carrying around vaccine in a plastic bag. I had heard about this incident from Dr. Ibrahim, so I knew that he had indeed been very upset. The peon said he was worried about his job, and he hoped a good word from me on his behalf would help him. I replied that the issue was not so much with him as with the supervisor who never got him a vaccine carrier in the first place and that as Dr. Ibrahim was senior to me, my word was unlikely to carry much weight in this situation. But the peon was adamant that I put in a good word for him. He didn't seem to consider that after his active involvement in lying in the business about the unvaccinated child, I might not be in a mood to help him.

When I finally got home, I felt a bit as if I had spent the day in a tank of sharks. As I remarked to Tanveer, the particularly frustrating thing was that the coverage in Sabazkot was actually very good (even if many of the children we saw were immunized only the day before, on the extra day given Sabazkot by the EDO). But I felt as if I had been manhandled for twelve hours and was exhausted from being on the defensive all day.

## Day 3

Tanveer and I headed back to the area of the city we had been supposed to check on the first day of monitoring. On our way, we called the area in charge who had stopped us from checking the other day.

When he picked up the phone, he said: "Oh, no, sorry, you can't do checking today. It's a national holiday." It was, in fact, a national holiday. However, the provincial office had placed a moratorium on holidays during polio campaigns. "There are no holidays in the world of polio," I said.

"But you were supposed to check the other area of the city and Sabaz-kot first," the area in charge protested.

I told him I had.

"When?" he asked, incredulous.

"Over the past two days," I replied.

"Oh," he said, apparently surprised. "You were working the last two days?"

However, he came about half an hour later, vaccine in hand, which was nice to see after Sabazkot. We went to the first area I planned to check, a small tent colony. The children in the tents were covered, but we found several missed children in nearby homes. Simply vaccinating the children in peace was not a possibility.

"Who knows why the mother decided to come out now!" lamented the lady health worker, a pleasant, petite woman who came out to meet us when we arrived. "I went to their house multiple times! She never came out before."

But the real storm came in the next area we checked, recently constructed brick houses placed almost randomly in a sea of dust baked by the hot sun. I checked a few houses with the area in charge. Tanveer was not with us, because he was trying to find a shady place to park the car, a challenge in this treeless area. At the third house I found a child whose mother insisted he was not vaccinated. The child had spent some time at his grandmother's house, the mother said, but she was sure he was not vaccinated there. I checked the child's hand; there was no finger marking.

During this discussion the area in charge and the lady health worker insisted repeatedly that the child was covered at his grandmother's. The area in charge could not possibly know this.

"Why isn't the finger marked, then?" I asked.

"The markers ran out of ink."

"Why didn't you get another marker?"

"We're not provided with any extra markers. And the markers all ran out of ink on the first day."

I wasn't in a mood to believe that, and regardless I had to mark the child as missed, based on parental report. I felt battered by the onslaught of argument by the area in charge and the lady health worker, and peeved that no finger marking had been done anywhere in this area, as that would have resolved the matter.

We were standing in the dusty street in this pool of ill feeling when Tanveer walked up. "Did you get the missed children in that house?" he asked.

Tanveer had been casually asking people about the vaccination status of people's children, just as a double check, as he walked toward us. At one of the houses I had already checked, Tanveer found several children of a guest; their mother said they had not been vaccinated. I had not seen the children when I had been at the door of the house, and the woman who lived there had not mentioned that she had any guests. I headed back to the house to speak to them again.

Now the area in charge was in full spate, screaming at Tanveer: "Who is this man, a driver, to go back over the houses that madam already checked? What are you trying to do? This is against the rules of checking!"

I tried to explain (though my patience was wearing extremely thin) that I was supposed to get information on every child in every household. "If I missed some by mistake," I said, "I am thankful to Tanveer for helping out."

The area in charge and the lady health worker continued the offensive, the area in charge telling me that according to how checking is supposed to be carried out, I was not allowed to go back into houses I had already checked. I was certainly not aware of any such rule.

"Just let me speak to the woman. Please," I said. I pressed my fingers against my head. When I went inside the house to speak to her, she said that her child was given drops last week; she thought, she said, we were asking about today. Since she could hear the screaming match taking place in front of her house, she may have decided that it was better to say her children had been vaccinated than to get involved in this mess.

As we left the house, the lady health worker, in hearing distance of several Pathan women in the road, started in on Pathans, an ethnic minority in this area of the Punjab. "They're so stupid," she said. "If they were vaccinated last week, they'll say no, we weren't vaccinated, because they want you to vaccinate them again. These Pathans, they don't understand anything."

I found one final child missed in that Union Council, in a fairly large house that the team had missed entirely. The mother was knowledgeable.

"They were supposed to be here on the twenty-fourth, twenty-fifth, and twenty-sixth, right? We were waiting," she said.

There was no chalking, so the fault of the team was pretty clear-cut. For once, we vaccinated the child without a fight or any screaming. As we walked away, I stepped in mud up to my ankle, and the family allowed me to use their bathroom to get the gunk off my foot.

We moved on to another Union Council, leaving the area in charge who had been with us thus far to enjoy his holiday. The area in charge of the next Union Council was Javed, a soft-spoken man who lived in another district and had never worked on a polio campaign before. When I asked why such a difficult Union Council without a single lady health worker would be assigned to someone who didn't know the area, lived fifty or sixty kilometers away, and had never worked on polio, Javed sighed.

Javed worked in a health post in Amirkhan near the border with the district where he lived. He had come into Kaifabad once to inquire about some back pay due him. There, planning for the polio rounds was going on. The area in charge assigned to this Union Council had refused to work, and so Javed was given a mandatory assignment to do duty here. He said he worked very hard on this polio campaign, not because he was interested in the work, but because he was terrified: he was told if missed children were found, he would lose his job. Javed had worked for the Health Department for twenty-four years, with just one year left before retirement. For him, assignment to this polio round was a giant and dangerous liability.

On Day 5 of the campaign, with whole swaths of his Union Council still uncovered, Javed had contacted someone higher up to get additional teams to help him cover it. That was why we hadn't been allowed to do checking on Sunday. Javed said he was fed up with polio. He said: "The zonal supervisor doesn't do anything. He doesn't actually do any checking. And he expects us to feed him lunch every day."

Amazingly, I found only two missed children in the four clusters I examined in this Union Council. Of course, Javed asked me to hide them. He also tried to bargain with me about which areas I would check, arguing that he should be the one to choose them. This approach was unsuccessful. The area was truly a difficult one, spread out with no good roads (my car took some serious whacks which would later require fixing), and all of it baking in the treeless sunshine.

Later in the day we moved on to the other Union Councils we were supposed to check that day. We could not reach anyone by phone: no area in charges, no zonal supervisors. But the maps of the area were good, so

Tanveer and I decided to work alone. Rather than being difficult, it was a pleasure and a luxury. When we found missed children, we simply marked them down and vaccinated them. There was no screaming, no argument, no fervent claims that people would lose their jobs.

In fact, at this point Tanveer and I began to take a perverse pleasure in every missed child we found. In retrospect, this attitude was perhaps unpardonable, but we had been driven over the edge. "I think I smell missed children over here," Tanveer would say, leading us gleefully down small dark alleyways. We joked that just to balance out all the falsified positive reports, we would create a falsified negative report of, say, 22 percent coverage in these Union Councils.

## Day 4

In the morning, I went to the district health office to turn in my monitoring results to Dr. Ibrahim. Perhaps because of all the argument, I felt uneasy about reporting my findings honestly. At the least, if people were fired based on my honest results, and others were not fired based on the falsified glowing reports of the campaign support persons, it would be unfair. Further, in any sampling technique like the one we were using for monitoring, some people would have poor results based on chance. I brought up my worries with Dr. Ibrahim and asked if he could bring these questions up with the EDO. Dr. Ibrahim did not seem as concerned as I was about people being fired. He opined that this round had a lot of problems, and that there would have to be some accountability.

As Tanveer and I were pulling out of the parking lot after our meeting with Dr. Ibrahim, we saw the campaign support person for the part of the city where Fahad worked. He and I were on good terms. We spoke in English. He said hello and asked about the results of my checking in the city, specifically about Fahad's area.

"They were guest children in that house of Fahad's that you checked," he said. "So it's unfair to count them against Fahad. He is a great worker and he's going to lose his job."

"No," I replied, "they weren't guest children. They lived there." (Whether they were guests or not, I was supposed to mark them down.) "However," I said, "I agree that it would be unfair to fire someone based on monitoring results alone, especially as some people had extra days and others did not—"

"Yes, yes, it would be unfair," the campaign support person interjected eagerly. "If he'd had extra time, those children would surely have been covered."

"I voiced those worries to Dr. Ibrahim," I said, "when I gave him my results."

"You already turned in your results?" the campaign support person said, clearly worried and disappointed.

"Yes," I said.

"And you counted those children against Fahad?"

"Yes."

"Madam," he said, "this is very bad. Because of this action of yours, Fahad is going to lose his job. If you had not taken this action, we would have kept one of our best workers."

## After the Campaign

The next day I got a call from Dr. Ibrahim. He was, he said, worried and frustrated after a long day of bargaining with the EDO. The EDO had agreed to four external monitors, but was still insisting that the district choose two of them. As these two would surely report 100 percent coverage, there was little added value to having them.

There was also a firestorm of complaint about how Dr. Ibrahim and I had done postcampaign monitoring. There were allegations that Dr. Ibrahim had visited forty to fifty houses in each area he checked, instead of the requisite seven. That this would have been humanly impossible in the time available was, I supposed, beside the point. There was also a complaint that I had not always checked houses "in a row," instead taking houses from both sides of a given street—a strange complaint, as which side of the street one chose to check should make no difference at all.

Tanveer brightened on hearing this last allegation. "I know where that's coming from," he said. "Remember that area in charge who was yelling at me about being a driver? He was complaining about that to me."

Then there were complaints about my status as a student: Where did she come from? Who gave her permission to work here? Why should we accept her monitoring results? What business does this Tanveer person have working with her? As this was my second time working in Kaifabad, I had neglected to procure the usual letter from the government's head of immunization in Islamabad. Getting a signature from him always required days and multiple visits, and it hadn't seemed worth the headache. Dr. Ibrahim said he told the EDO that I was introduced prior to the campaign, that the EDO was encouraging, and that if the district had required additional documentation that would have been the time to request it.

I discussed this issue with the Islamabad office. They felt that getting a letter now would cause more trouble than it was worth. If the district didn't want to accept my results, they pointed out, I could share my observations with them informally. They were surprised that the district was raising such a hue and cry about my results when I was reporting 96 percent coverage—a perfectly acceptable number. But, they said, this was not the first time such problems had arisen in Kaifabad. One person noted that a high-ranking official in Kaifabad was "one of the best in the Punjab" but also "head of the mafia."

Dr. Ibrahim's driver, a WHO employee, was accused of bringing Dr. Ibrahim to the most difficult, uncovered areas on purpose—which was, in fact, where monitors were instructed to go. There was also a complaint by some campaign support persons that Dr. Ibrahim wouldn't let them check four Union Councils per day in rural areas. This was surprising, as while doing only three Union Councils in rural areas had initially been my idea, it was enthusiastically endorsed by all campaign support persons present—who had, in fact, tried to make additional cuts in their own workloads.

As Dr. Ibrahim observed, none of the complaints was substantive. It seemed to me that all of them had the same goal: to punish Dr. Ibrahim for being too proactive during the campaign and to prevent him from working in Kaifabad in the future. I felt bad for Dr. Ibrahim because, though at times he may have come on strong, he worked hard and in good faith.

I'm not sure how, but the four external monitors that Dr. Ibrahim originally wanted were assigned to the district after all. Combined with the other postcampaign monitoring results, the overall official coverage number for the district was 98 percent of all children under five. This high number was the result of eight or nine of the campaign support persons reporting coverage of 100 or 99.9 percent, a practically impossible circumstance. Realistic reports came from Dr. Ibrahim, Dr. Ahmed, a couple of campaign support persons, and some (though not all) of the external monitors. Coverage of 98 percent is very good. However, the district leadership remained upset; they coveted their usual 99 percent coverage rate. The WHO official who received the numbers shrugged his shoulders. "I don't care," he said. "Anything above 95 is fine as far as I am concerned."

I mentioned to the official my feeling that this brouhaha may have been a way of getting back at Dr. Ibrahim for finding too many problems.

The official nodded. He said that for that reason, foreign consultants are purposely assigned to new districts every five months or so. He mentioned that people assigned to a new district were likely to go after problems proactively, but after some time in a given district, the foreign consultants often felt accountable for the results there and began defending the quality of the work rather than finding problems.

About a month later, Tanveer told me he had seen Fahad. "He was carrying a vaccine carrier in his area," he said.

"So he wasn't fired?" I asked.

"Nope. Apparently not."

## Public Buses

Reema is a lady health worker who lives in a small village
outside Kaifabad. I visit her in the very early spring, when the
mustard is in bloom; the fields around the cluster of cement
buildings that make up her village are brilliant yellow. Reema's
supervisor leads me up the narrow, muddy alleyway to her
house. After warmly welcoming her supervisor, who leaves
after introducing us, Reema invites me into the formal part
of the house, a dark room with cement walls and floors. We
sit on a wooden couch with hand-embroidered covers on
its foam cushions. Reema serves Mountain Dew in chipped
glasses and talks about her work on polio campaigns.

> When you consider that we go door-to-door, our pay
> is nothing. But thinking of God [_khudā ko nazar nazar
> rakh-kar_], we say we've left our house to work, we should
> do our duty well. . . . The problem comes when we have
> to work in areas we don't know well. We know our own
> areas, so covering all the children there is easy. You know
> whether there are children in a certain house, right?
> When we go to other areas, that's when problems come
> up. People don't know you, you don't know whether there
> are children in the house or not, and then you are with
> another lady health worker, both women. If there was a
> man with us, then we wouldn't be frightened.
>   That's why all the lady health workers say we don't
> make nearly enough money for as hard as we work. . . .
> Even refreshments, we get sometimes and sometimes not.
> And then our monthly pay, the 1900 rupees [about $30],
> it doesn't come every month, it doesn't come regularly, it
> doesn't come on time. . . .

We have to work all day long for five or six days, and then there are still problems [*pher bhī yih pareshāni hojati hai*]. We do the best job we can [*kisi jagah apnī taraf-se nahin choṛte*]. Then, when later the people come to check our work they make a fuss [*shor kartehein*] and say, "You didn't do good work, we found a missed child here." This creates huge difficulties for us.

Look, the next campaign is in the summer—that one will be tough. In that much heat, your sweat never dries. But what can I do—I have to work, I have to answer to my supervisor every evening, I have to give reports to *his* supervisor. . . .

To get to some of the places where I work during polio days, I have to change buses twice. I have to change a bus just to get to the basic health unit where I go every evening to give my report and every morning to pick up the day's vaccine. Look, those bus fares add up. Every day it costs me 20 or 30 rupees [50 cents]. . . . Think, every day going to the basic health unit to get vaccine takes time, it takes bus fare, and then you have to work the rest of the day.

Do something about the pay—some of us are very poor. My husband had an accident and broke his leg— for ten months he hasn't really worked.

# CHAPTER 4

# Kaifabad

TANVEER AND I SPOKE several times about what drove us crazy during monitoring in Kaifabad and in other districts we visited. "The thing is," one of us would say, "that if people working in Kaifabad spent half as much energy planning and executing a good campaign as they did evading the monitors, the vaccination coverage would be perfect." We would shake our heads. "It's so stupid."

While our frustration was real, our evaluation was unfair. Government employees working on polio eradication at the district level in Pakistan were not stupid. Making sense of their behavior is important, because ultimately the quality of work at the ground level determines whether polio eradication is possible.

## Everyday Resistance

In his excellent book *Weapons of the Weak*, James C. Scott describes "everyday forms of peasant resistance":

> Most forms of this struggle stop well short of outright collective defiance. Here I have in mind the ordinary weapons of relatively powerless groups: foot dragging, dissimulation, desertion, false compliance, pilfering, feigned ignorance, slander, arson, sabotage, and so on. These Brechtian—or Schweikian—forms of class struggle have certain features in common. They require little or no coordination or planning; they make use of implicit understandings and informal networks; they often represent a form of individual self-help; they typically avoid any direct, symbolic confrontation with authority. To understand these commonplace forms of resistance is to understand much of what the peasantry has historically done to defend its interests against both conservative and progressive orders. It is my guess that just such kinds of resistance are often the most significant and the most effective over the long run. . . .

> Their individual acts of foot dragging and evasion, reinforced by a ven-
> erable popular culture of resistance and multiplied many thousand-fold,
> may, in the end, make an utter shambles of the policies dreamed up by
> their would-be superiors in the capital. (Scott 1985, xvi–xvii)

The behavior of people working at the ground level of the Polio Eradication Initiative makes sense when it is approached in terms of Scott's for-
mulation of everyday resistance. District employees resisted the directives
of their superiors in a number of ways, including refusal to work, falsification, what is normally referred to as "corruption," false compliance, and
direct confrontation.

### Refusal to Work

One of the clearest forms of resistance to superiors is the strike. Government health employees in Pakistan are not unionized, and in a context
of high unemployment one would not expect strikes to be common in
the Polio Eradication Initiative. However, at least one quite limited strike
did occur. Through an administrative miscommunication, workers in one
district were overpaid for training during one campaign. By the next campaign, the mistake had been corrected and the workers were back to being
paid fifty cents for training. Their response was to refuse to attend. Polio eradication planners noted in their internal campaign report that they
would, in the future, avoid "gathering all supervisors in one or two places
to conduct training there and likewise to avoid calling for strike."

Much more common than strikes were less-organized refusals to work
on polio. Finding people, especially women, to do the door-to-door vaccination was an ongoing problem in some districts. In one district, less than
half the lady health workers on the books worked on polio campaigns. In
another, difficulties in obtaining volunteers to work as vaccinators were so
severe that the campaign was routinely extended from three days to nine
or twelve days so that the limited workforce could cover the city.

Even those who agreed to work on campaigns might not perform all
the tasks expected of them. This was a particular problem with teams
working at transit points, who were supposed to vaccinate all children that
came by. As they did not have a fixed area that could be checked, it was
easy for them to take time off from work. Supervisors who arrived to find
them not at their posts were told they had just left for a moment to go to
the bathroom, or to get a drink of water, or to pray. (Transit-point workers

were notorious for praying even at times of the day when no prayer was requisite.)

Another ongoing problem was teams' recording of "missed children." At each house teams visited, they were supposed to ask whether any children were not at home, record the names and ages of those children, and return to the house during catch-up days to vaccinate them. This entailed quite a bit of work and was a step team members were wont to skip. As covering missed children was essential to achieving a rate of vaccination coverage high enough to interrupt polio transmission, this was a critical omission.

In poorly run districts, supervisors too shirked their duty. In one district I was monitoring, I spent the better part of a day trying to find one area in charge who had left a note saying that he was checking teams in a remote part of his area and that there might not be a cell-phone signal there. Tanveer and I drove to that area, which was completely uninhabited—there were no children, and thus no need for teams—but in fact had excellent cell-phone coverage. Later, we were told that the man in question had a "*very* old cell phone," which explained why he couldn't get a signal in the areas where he was checking nonexistent teams vaccinating nonexistent populations. The supervisors in Sabazkot described in Chapter 3, who arrived late, didn't have vaccine, and claimed to vaccinate children when they had not, are a less extreme example of the same type of behavior. And this behavior was not limited to lower-level supervisors; one doctor told me that campaign support persons "don't work half the time—if it's raining they just sort of phone in." In the worst-performing districts, EDOs too would not attend evening meetings.

## Falsification and Lying

Tied to refusing to work was falsifying the requisite records to make it appear that work had been done (see Chapter 3 for several examples). Teams could chalk the next day's date on a house if they did their work ahead of time, or mark a house as containing no children if no one was home and they did not want to have to return another day. Much more widespread than this sort of falsification on the team level was falsification of monitoring results, an activity that involved participants from the teams up to the campaign support persons and perhaps the district leadership.

The comment by Javed asserting that his zonal supervisor "doesn't actually do any checking, and he expects us to feed him lunch every day" reveals one way of falsifying monitoring results. Rather than go door-to-door as he was supposed to do, Javed noted, his zonal supervisor copied Javed's own door-to-door monitoring results. Insofar as those numbers were good, this worked in Javed's favor. In return, Javed was expected to purchase lunch for his supervisor.

A similar pattern shows up in the repeated appeals to my humanity as a superior to overlook the mistakes of those I was supervising. I was also, often unwittingly, on the receiving end of gifts of food and hospitality. At some point during each day of work, lunch was inevitable. Lunch was an activity I looked forward to with some trepidation. Those whose work I was evaluating unfailingly insisted on paying for my lunch, which they could often ill afford. Further, once I had accepted a free lunch, I found that expectations that I would cover up any mistakes were generally heightened. Once I had accepted hospitality, become a guest and a friend, it was more difficult for me to fulfill my role as evaluator. Attempts on my part to pay for everyone's lunch were often stoutly resisted on the grounds that they would be hurt were I to resist their hospitality. (In Pakistan, splitting checks is unheard of.) Tanveer and I would resort to elaborate schemes, for instance, he would pretend to get up and go to the bathroom during the meal and surreptitiously pay the bill. Even this did not always work, as our would-be hosts had usually warned restaurant staff not to let us pay. In Marcel Mauss's terms, I had an "obligation to receive," and I would be expected to give something in return—namely, a positive evaluation (Mauss 1967).

Both Javed and I were caught in relationships of reciprocity in which lunches or hospitality were extended to superiors, and in return the short-comings of inferiors were overlooked. As my use of the words "superiors" and "inferiors" implies, these relationships were not equal ones. They were characterized by inequality as well as reciprocity, relationships commonly referred to as "patron-client" (Foster 1963; Weingrod 1968). Again, James C. Scott provides a useful definition: "The patron-client relationship—an exchange relationship between roles—may be defined as a special case of dyadic (two-person) ties involving a largely instrumental friendship in which an individual of higher socioeconomic status (patron) uses his own influence and resources to provide protection or benefits, or both, for a person of lower status (client) who, for his part, reciprocates by offering general support and assistance, including personal services, to the patron" (Scott 1972, 92).

Scholars have made two observations about patron-client relationships that illuminate the reasons for their importance in the context of the Pakistani health bureaucracy. The first is that they tend to be found in situations where other systems of authority are unpredictable (Foster 1963). Systems of accountability were often perceived as capricious by people low in the hierarchy of the Pakistani health bureaucracy; here, patron-client relationships provided low-level employees like lady health workers and areas in charge, as well as their supervisors, with a "personal security mechanism" in an uncertain context (Scott 1972, 102).[1]

The second characteristic of patron-client relationships relevant to our discussion of resistance is that they often "undermine the formal structure of authority" (Scott 1972, 92). Myriad patron-client relationships in the Pakistani health system melded into a system quite effective at obscuring areas of poor work. In fact, the patron-client system was so good at covering up red areas of low vaccination coverage that by 2006, incidence of reported red areas did not correlate, as it should have, with poliovirus circulation. Several years earlier, red areas had been a strong predictor of likely polio cases; the negative attention given red areas apparently resulted in attempts to cover them up (as in the case of Fahad described earlier). Evidently the majority of such attempts were successful.

While patron-client relationships were ubiquitous in the Pakistani health system, even those who participated in them approached them with some ambivalence.[2] The following accusations were leveled by a subordinate against a WHO district-level official in a letter to WHO headquarters in Islamabad: "He is a bewildered and misdirected personality at odds with every one in the district and behaving as a master. His attitude to the district authorities is also not appreciable. He used to take gifts from CSPs [campaign support persons] and others and lunch/dinner from poor vaccinators."

I too received justifiable criticism. When I was assigned to do monitoring in Malakot in an earlier campaign in Kaifabad, on the third day everything looked very good, but we mostly saw only what we were shown. The zonal supervisor traveling with us called teams and area in charges as we approached: "Be ready—a team of foreigners has come for checking." Where we did find problems, the explanation was always that these were areas slated to be covered later in the day. As always, as we traveled, we accumulated layers of supervisors. At one point there were seven of us traveling together.

Oranges were in season in Malakot, and at one point the campaign support person traveling with us asked Tanveer to stop. He jumped out of the car and rapidly purchased a large crate of oranges at a roadside stand, which he placed in my trunk. Once it became clear that the oranges were a gift for me, we were well down the road and returning them seemed impracticable. How would I get the campaign support person to take the money back?

About a month later I was back in Malakot interviewing lady health workers. I spoke to a doctor who worked for the Health Department, who asked if I had worked on the previous campaign. I said yes. "I heard about you," he said. "You came as far as the orange stand, let them buy you oranges, and turned around." My only defense—ignorance—was a weak one.

## Corruption

While many would—and did—view the instances of patron-clientism described here as "corrupt," I am hesitant to use that term because, as in the case of my interactions with Fahad in the last chapter, engaging in behavior that would protect the jobs of subordinates often seemed a moral course of action (see also Smith 2001; Werner 2000). However, I am willing to label as "corruption" instances in which people siphoned money from the Polio Eradication Initiative for purely personal gain.[3]

Such instances were relatively rare. Once I came across an area in charge who had vastly overestimated the number of children in the area he was responsible for and then created phantom teams to cover the nonexistent children so that he might pocket the money allocated for these teams. But given the low rate of pay for teams, the amount the area in charge gained from this elaborate exercise in falsification was less than thirty dollars.[4]

Given the relatively small amounts of money involved, monetary corruption did not significantly impact the trajectory of the Polio Eradication Initiative. The majority of instances I was aware of, like the one described here, were on the level of petty pilfering. The extremely high levels of supervision in the Polio Eradication Initiative made large-scale diversion of funds difficult. (On several occasions, WHO and UNICEF employees in Islamabad attributed obstructive behavior by some districts' politicians or government health employees to their frustration that they could not get their hands on polio money.) But insofar as such small-scale corruption fits into the constellation of activities that constitute resistance, it is significant. And as the number of children under five in Pakistan reported to Polio Eradication Initiative planners by districts was significantly higher than that recorded in the national census, practices like the one described here probably were not uncommon.[5]

## False Compliance

On one occasion, a midlevel government official invited a foreign WHO employee to speak to officials in her area about the importance of polio eradication. Pleased at the seeming collaboration from an area of the country that had always been difficult, the WHO employee gladly made the trip.

When he arrived at the meeting, the government official spoke to the others assembled in Urdu. She indicated the WHO employee, who could not understand her words. "Listen to him politely," she is reported to have said, "but you can do whatever you want."

In this case and in others, government officials made only a show of being compliant and supportive of polio eradication. Here, the supervisor made explicit to her subordinates that although she expected them to appear interested in what WHO leadership had to say, they did not have to take the actions that the WHO was suggesting.

## Direct Confrontation

While false compliance was common and indicated that the Polio Eradication Initiative wielded at least enough power to ensure discursive commitment to polio eradication, in certain rare contexts Polio Eradication Initiative officials faced direct insubordination.[6] The cases I observed were generally when people felt would-be superiors were stepping out of bounds, and when those people had little real authority.

For example, I worked in one district with another foreign consultant, not a WHO employee but a volunteer deployed by CDC from another South Asian country.[7] This man was trying to get vaccinators in the district in question to standardize their recording of nonpolio, routine immunizations.

"You shouldn't be giving vaccine to children over one year old," the foreigner said.

"You wouldn't give vaccine to an unvaccinated two-year-old?" a vaccinator asked, in a challenging sort of way.

"We wouldn't," said the foreigner sternly.

"We are," the vaccinator shot back.

In this case of direct insubordination, the foreigner had, it appeared to his subordinates, overstepped his bounds by dealing with issues other than polio. The value of his advice was also questionable. In this context, the subordinate was bold enough to engage in direct, confrontational resistance.

### *Other Strategies of Resistance*

The methods of resistance listed so far do not come near exhausting the strategies employed by people working on polio in various times and places. A number of additional strategies were used in Kaifabad, as we have seen. Grumbling ("Whatever you say, madam") was a common strategy, a way of expressing discontent without the appearance of insubordination (Scott 1990). Bargaining ("We'll accept four outside evaluators, but we get to choose two") was another. Simple evasion was also effective, as in the case of a team of lady health workers who ducked into an alleyway when they saw me coming.

Strategies of resistance district workers employed were multiple, diffuse, and unorganized. Taken together, however, they could, from the perspective of a foreign consultant, form a nearly impenetrable shield. While they were not planned in a coordinated way, their effectiveness as a whole was impressive. Were it not for these strategies of resistance, polio would likely have been eradicated in Pakistan years ago.

## Corruption versus Resistance

In anthropological literature, at least, "resistance" is often infused with a positive valence, "corruption" rarely. Some, then, might view grouping "corruption" with "resistance" as romanticizing corruption. In the case of the Polio Eradication Initiative, I would not argue that resistance was necessarily a positive social force. But beyond that simple assertion, my approach to "corruption"—and its fraught relation with resistance—bears some explanation.

There are two major positions in an ongoing debate about the impact of corruption on development.[8] Let's call them the "corruption blocks development" thesis and the "corruption doesn't matter" thesis.

A proponent of the corruption-blocks-development thesis is Thomas Friedman, who wrote in the 2005 best seller *The World Is Flat:* "These rural Indians understood, at gut level, exactly why it was not happening for them: because local governments in India have become so eaten away by corruption and mismanagement that they cannot deliver to the poor the schools and infrastructure they need to get a fair share of the pie"

(383). Similarly, the prominent anticorruption NGO Transparency International argued that "it is now a fairly established fact that corruption is severely undermining development objectives in South Asian countries by hindering economic growth, reducing efficiency, acting as a disincentive to potential investors and, above all, by diverting critical resources meant for poverty alleviation" (Transparency International 2002, 5). Given that Transparency International ranks Pakistan in the top quartile for corruption among the world's countries (Transparency International 2008), and that in one of their surveys 96 percent of respondents reported encountering corruption in the Pakistani health sector (ibid., 2002, 2), on the surface it is plausible that corruption could be the culprit in polio eradication's difficulties.[9]

And polio eradication was not free from corruption. But, as I believe, if "corruption" refers to the siphoning off of money, it happened on such a small scale that of itself it was almost certainly not the reason for the difficulties the project faced.

The situation changes a bit if one considers the patron-client relations described earlier to be corruption, as they likely had a somewhat larger impact on the trajectory of polio eradication. But if one accepts Transparency International's own definition of corruption as "the misuse of entrusted power for private gain," it is not at all clear that patron-client relationships, and the falsification they entail, constitute corruption.[10] What makes patron-client relationships so tricky from the perspective of a supervisor— and what likely contributes to making them so pervasive—is that, in the context of poor job security, protecting a subordinate from being fired often appears a moral course of action. The main benefits a patron receives from a patron-client relationship are often respect and deference, not material items one can refuse (Wolf 1966). While it is true that the lunches I consumed constituted private gain, I would have preferred to pay for them myself.

Regardless of whether one considers patron-client relationships to constitute corruption, however, their impact on the trajectory of polio eradication, while more considerable than that of monetary corruption, was probably not by itself sufficient to stymie the project. This brings us to the corruption-doesn't-matter thesis, whose most visible proponent is probably the economist Jeffrey Sachs. In the 2005 best-selling *End of Poverty*, Sachs wrote: "If the poor are poor because they are lazy or their governments are corrupt, how could global cooperation help? Fortunately, these common beliefs are misconceptions, only a small part of the explanation, if at all, of why the poor are poor. I have noted repeatedly that in all corners of the world, the poor face structural challenges that keep them from getting even their first foot on the ladder of development" (226). Sachs's approach is appealing in its refusal to blame the failures of development projects on the poor or their culture rather than on structural factors.[11] Sachs is correct too in noting that corruption per se is no more than a miniscule piece of the explanation of why development is not happening in many parts of the world, and is not sufficient to explain the failure of many development projects.

But I am not prepared to disregard the impact of corruption entirely. If corruption did not have a significant impact on the trajectory of polio eradication on its own, neither did the occasional strike, or grumbling by employees, or the odd act of insubordination. However, these strategies of resistance, taken together, coalesced into something that could derail planners' objectives.

In the context of polio eradication, acts of corruption functioned in much the same way as other acts of resistance did. However, while a strike is an act of resisting the demands of one's superiors on ideological grounds, pocketing money might have to do more with opportunism than with ideological opposition, which raises the question of motive. Once again, James C. Scott offers a useful perspective:

> The problem lies in what is a misleading, sterile, and sociologically naïve insistence upon distinguishing "self-indulgent," individual acts, on the one hand, from presumably "principled," selfless, collective actions, on the other, and excluding the former from the category of *real* resistance. . . . To ignore the self-interested element in peasant resistance is to ignore the determinate context not only of peasant politics, but of most lower-class politics. It is precisely the fusion of self-interest and resistance that is the vital force animating the resistance of peasants and proletarians. . . . To require of lower-class resistance that it somehow be "principled" or "selfless" is not only utopian and a slander on the moral status of fundamental material needs; it is, more fundamentally, a misconstruction of the basis of class struggle, which is, first and foremost, a struggle over the appropriation of work, production, property, and taxes. (Scott 1985, 295)

Scott's argument applies in the case of corruption in the Polio Eradication Initiative. Corruption fits neatly into patterns of resistance insofar as it was, like the other forms of resistance carried out by people at the lowest level of the polio eradication hierarchy, in large part about how much work could be expected from people at a rate of pay insufficient to fill their children's bellies. My argument here is not necessarily that pilfering from the Polio Eradication Initiative, or other acts of resistance that employees engaged in, were virtuous. It is simply that these acts, and their significant effects in making polio eradication very difficult to achieve, can be understood as part of a matrix of resistance.

## Why Resist?

Workers in Pakistani districts were not resisting the achievement of polio eradication per se. No one desired the ongoing paralysis of children. Workers I spoke to were unanimous in their opinion that vaccinating children against polio was a moral act. The reasons that people resisted varied slightly depending on their position in the Health Department hierarchy.

### Lady Health Workers and Area in Charges: Pay and Respect

Lady health workers were nearly unanimous in their complaints over one issue: pay. They received a salary of about thirty dollars a month for their part-time work for the Health Department; they received an additional two dollars a day for campaign days and fifty cents for attending training. The women I interviewed nearly all felt that the pay was much too low when one considered the work they had to do. This complaint applied both to the pay for polio campaigns and to their general salaries as lady health workers. The few women I spoke to who did not complain about pay for polio work were those who held higher posts and whose pay was above a hundred dollars per month. Thus complaints about low pay for polio days were tied to overall dissatisfaction with salary.

Many of the women I interviewed were angry about their low pay. It made them feel disrespected and undervalued, especially when, as they pointed out, the success or failure of polio eradication depends on their work. Compounding the sense of disrespect related to pay was that most lady health workers knew that campaign support persons, who were doctors, earned around seventeen dollars per day. That the services of campaign support persons should be valued so highly while their own remuneration was minimal was experienced as a slight.

Several women I interviewed had husbands who earned little or nothing and were attempting to support their families through their work as lady health workers. However, their pay, even when combined with polio pay, was not nearly enough to provide anything of substance for their families. One focus group discussed this issue:

> Lady health worker 1: It's true that when someone asks how much we make we are ashamed, we don't tell the truth, we just say it's enough to live on.
> Lady health worker 2: Now, they did a good thing by raising the pay for polio days from 400 to 600 rupees [from about $7 to about $10 for five days of work]. But we get it so late. When Allah is happy, then we get paid.
> Lady health worker 3: And the money for meetings—we don't always get it. Sometimes.
> LHW 1: Only sometimes and then only very little.
> LHW 2: Here in Pakistan if an unskilled laborer works from eight in the morning to four in the afternoon he will get 200 rupees [$3.50] per day. This 120 rupees [$2] per day is not enough; we have to go door-to-door. To get to other villages we have to pay bus fare—to the center and to the villages; the money goes in the bus fare. We do this work because, okay, it's related to our work as a lady health worker, so we should do it.

Women I spoke to in individual interviews were also upset about pay:

> Pay is very low; they might as well not pay us at all. Then they say we don't work hard enough.

> Every day we spend twenty or thirty rupees [fifty cents] on transportation. Look, every day there is a meeting, and we have to pay bus fare for that. Then we pick up the vaccine and that same bus fare. . . . On Day 5 when we submit our rechecking report, we have to spend the bus fare again. Think about it: for all those days, daily going to the health post and picking up the vaccine takes time, it takes bus fare, and then of course there is the actual work of vaccination to be done—it's a big problem.

> You can spend millions of rupees from the top, you can do anything from the top, but practically we have to do the work. If you don't respect us, we won't do good work.

All the workers say our pay is so low, they say who knows how much money is coming to us from above, and how much we actually get.

As did the woman in the final quote, many lady health workers suspected—incorrectly—that their superiors were skimming off some of their pay. Their reasoning was that a huge international program like the Polio Eradication Initiative would probably not pay them so little. But in fact they were receiving the full amount allocated to them.[12]

Lady health workers also felt disrespected by upper-level supervisors; they felt that while good work was not appreciated, mistakes were blown out of proportion. One of the focus groups of lady health workers discussed this issue:

> Lady health worker 1: The vaccinators [area in charges] are good, but the people who come for checking put way too much pressure on the vaccinators and way too much pressure on us.
>
> Lady health worker 2: We're human; we make mistakes. If there's some small mistake, they turn it into this big thing, and where there is good work, they don't say anything or they ignore it.
>
> LHW 1: And then they tell people in Kaifabad, and we have to go to Kaifabad so many times . . .
>
> LHW 2: Take this woman here. She has always done good work. Last month she had an accident and she told her vaccinator about it and that she couldn't work. Still there was a complaint lodged against her and she got a termination letter. She went to Kaifabad and they reinstated her but they cut one month of pay—that's no way to treat someone.
>
> LHW 1: They should cooperate with us at least a little.
>
> LHW 3: The vaccinators [area in charges] are good. But the people in Kaifabad who sit on chairs all day . . . if some child is missed—after all we are the children of humans, we make mistakes, anyone can make a mistake. Tell the Kaifabad team: deal gently with us, don't terminate us or cut off pay so immediately.
>
> LHW 4: They stop people's pay.
>
> LHW 3: They stop one, two months of pay, and then you have to go to Kaifabad how many times to get your pay reinstated.

Lady health workers did not question the value of immunizing children. But they were underpaid and they felt disrespected. Most of them were working because they were in need of money, but they were receiving very little. The core ground-level workforce of the Polio Eradication Initiative was at best disgruntled and at worst irate.

Area in charges were concerned largely about the same issues as lady health workers: pay and respect. However, area in charges were paid somewhat better than lady health workers. They were usually drawn from a class of workers that made $100 a month or somewhat more, and their additional pay on polio days was about $2.40 a day. They were generally not angry about pay in the way that lady health workers were, yet several noted that they usually spent their polio pay on incentives for their team members in the course of their work: "Two samosas for each team member when I visit them make them happy, make them feel appreciated," one explained to me.

Area in charges were also subject to the whims of their supervisors and expected to show respect, as one described to me:

> Some time ago another madam came to the evening meetings in Kaifabad. She only spoke a little Urdu. . . . She started talking to us in English. One of our friends is a vaccinator over in Amirkhan. He only studied to eighth class, is a great worker, but he doesn't know when to shut up. He stood up in protest: "Please, get someone who can talk in Punjabi, or at least Urdu!" Later he got in trouble with the EDO: "Why did you disrespect her?"

Polio eradication leadership, to this area in charge, was by turns unintelligible (the foreign consultant) and capricious (the EDO). If area in charges as a group could not, like lady health workers, be characterized as angry, polio campaigns often seemed to area in charges like a giant pain with little benefit. Once I was with several area in charges when we were served *zamzam*, holy water from Mecca. We turned toward Mecca and drank the small glasses of water while offering a prayer. "Pray that polio will be eradicated," said one area in charge. "Then we won't have to keep on doing this any more [*jān ćhūt-jāegi*]."

### District Leadership: An Unrealistic Goal with Few Benefits

The position of the district leadership—the EDO and those who worked with him—was in many ways more complicated than that of the lady health workers, for it involved them in contradictory roles. Sometimes they exerted power over lower-level workers to carry out the demands of the Polio Eradication Initiative, and at other times they resisted those same demands coming from WHO (cf. Chandavarkar 1991).

Polio eradication activities took a lot of time and energy, which inevitably left less time to focus on other health goals. Because polio campaigns are part of an eradication strategy, participation was mandated for each district; clearly, the strategy would not be effective if some districts could opt out. But many people in district leadership felt that polio eradication campaigns were not the best use of time.

Some government officials resented the large amounts of money that UN agencies felt free to spend. At one campaign inauguration, I witnessed the following exchange between a government official (not in the Health Department) and a UNICEF employee, as glossy End Polio planners and pins were being passed out to everyone in attendance:

> Government official: How much do you pay for rent for your office?
> UNICEF employee: I don't know.
> Government official: Did you guys print these planners?
> UNICEF employee: Yes.
> Government official: How much did you spend for each one?
> UNICEF employee: I don't know.
> Government official: Did you guys make these badges [pins]?
> UNICEF employee: Yes.
> Government official: How much did you spend for each one?
> UNICEF employee: I don't know.

The government official's implication was clear: UNICEF is a money-wasting machine.

But resistance, for district leadership, was primarily not about pay or resources but about ideology (cf. Rogers 1991). If belief in eradication as a strategy is akin to a religion, as I have argued, there were plenty of doubters in Pakistani districts. Many people in district leadership felt that if polio had not been eradicated after nearly ten years of campaigns in Pakistan, it never would be. One high-level district official in Kaifabad opined that routine immunizations had been "suffering" because manpower was always diverted for polio campaigns. "Polio will not be eradicated," he told me. Similarly, I attended one meeting where an EDO told area in charges: "Polio does interfere with routine EPI work because it takes so much time. We'll do campaigns, though, because WHO and the donor agencies want it that way, and it's okay."[13]

District leadership was pressed harder and harder with each passing year to be committed to polio eradication, a goal many believed to be un-realistic and to detract from more pressing issues such as low levels of rou-tine immunization. That nominal district health leaders could not make decisions on priorities themselves, and had to constantly chase after the latest global health fad advocated by WHO, probably rankled. Further, achieving eradication would bring questionable political benefits.

In the administrative structure that Pakistan inherited from the British Raj, policy was set by secretariats in the capital while administration of everyday duties was the responsibility of the district administration (Islam 2004). In this system, district-level bureaucracies were top-down, leaving them unaccountable to people living in the district in question (Cheema, Khwaja, and Qadir 2005). In 2001–2002, Musharraf implemented a far-reaching program of decentralization, creating new local governments and making EDOs accountable to the new district elected official, the *nazim*, in addition to the provincial or district governments (Keefer, Narayan, and Vishwanath 2003). EDOs are now accountable to two masters, as most policy decisions and funding still come from Islamabad, but the *nazim* can request the transfer of an EDO he is unhappy with.[14]

This system significantly weakened the power of the federal govern-ment to put pressure on EDOs and drew the EDOs into politics at the district level.[15] The extent of the EDO's involvement in local politics in a place like Kaifabad remained opaque to me, as it did to most other foreign consultants, but I was often under the impression that there were back-stage maneuverings I did not understand. Anecdotes of *nazims* exerting pressure on EDOs to make political appointments, even down to the level of lady health worker, were in wide circulation.[16]

Decentralization was not uniformly bad for health outcomes. Some important indicators, such as the percentage of doctors showing up for work at rural health posts, have improved dramatically since 2000.[17] This indicates that local demand for health services can result in political pres-sure and improvement in service delivery. Therefore, if a large proportion of the Pakistani population was passionate about polio, as the U.S. popu-lation was in the 1950s, there might be political pressure for eradication activities to be of the highest quality. But there was not. Thus, for an EDO to spend two weeks focusing on polio eradication at the expense of other projects as many as eight times a year could be a frustrating imperative.

Pakistanis as a whole were not opposed to polio immunization.[18] When the immunization teams came to their houses, almost everyone gave drops to their children. But this acceptance was mostly passive: it was the rare parent who brought a child to the health post to get additional doses of vaccine if the child was missed during the campaign.[19] And given the large and very pressing problems facing the nation, polio coverage certainly did not rate as an election issue anywhere in Pakistan.

Historian James Colgrove notes that in the United States in the early 1900s, polio "sparked a popular terror far out of proportion to the number of deaths it caused" (Colgrove 2006, 114; Oshinsky 2005). This is not the case in Pakistan or in many other poor countries, largely because of differences in the epidemiology of poliovirus in a place like the United States and in a place like Pakistan. Prior to the development of polio vaccines, in wealthy industrialized countries with temperate climates, polio was an epidemic disease, sweeping through the population, often in the summer, and paralyzing relatively large numbers of people at once, older children and adults as well as infants. In poor countries like Pakistan with scant sanitation infrastructures and warm climates, polio's transmission is very different. In these areas (and in Europe prior to around 1850), polio is an endemic disease, occurring at a constant level rather than in epidemic waves and affecting mostly infants (Smallman-Raynor et al. 2006).[20] Epidemics are more likely to inspire terror than are diseases that occur constantly at low levels. Even in the United States, once polio vaccination became available and the threat of epidemic less immediate, public enthusiasm for vaccination waned quickly (Colgrove 2006).

Further, with the introduction of polio immunization in poor countries, the burden of disease from polio shifts almost entirely to the poor (Risi 1997). As with the frustrating headmaster in Kaifabad, the elites that drive priorities in Pakistan felt—accurately, in fact—that polio was not a disease likely to strike their children.[21] Without great concern over polio on the part of elites, it was unlikely to become a political priority.

Yet, some planners in Geneva continued to insist in their optimism that with better social mobilization, polio could become a political issue in Pakistan. A high-level WHO official who visited Islamabad told Pakistani WHO employees that they had to create popular demand for polio immunization, which in a democracy would naturally lead to the quality of polio campaigns being a political priority. With limited control over districts, planners in Geneva continued to wait in vain for political commitment that never materialized—and that never would. In the absence of such commitment, they resorted to other techniques to put pressure on districts.

## Resistance and Power

Acts of resistance do not exist in a vacuum. When people resist, they are resisting something (or someone) with power over them. Several scholars have suggested that identifying acts of resistance can help pin down that nebulous thing called power. Foucault suggests "using this resistance as a chemical catalyst so as to bring to light power relations, locate their position, and find out their point of application and the methods used" (Foucault 1982, 780). Lila Abu-Lughod notes usefully that such an approach leads away from a romanticization of acts of resistance as "signs of human freedom" and toward an understanding that people resist because they are "caught up" in webs of power relations (Abu-Lughod 1990b). Douglas Haynes and Gyan Prakash note further that power and resistance are "constantly intermeshed," not separable entities but continually acting on and shaping one another (Haynes and Prakash 1992, 19). Acts of power and of resistance are mutually constitutive. If we are to speak of everyday techniques of resistance, then it is useful too to examine everyday techniques of power. Each shapes the other. The everyday acts of power used by district-level supervisors in the Polio Eradication Initiative will be the focus of the next section.

In the context of the district-level interactions on which I will focus here, Weber's definition of power as "the probability that one actor within a social relationship will be in a position to carry out his own will despite resistance" is useful (Weber 1978, 53). This dyadic model of power and resistance leaves out "structural power" (Barrett 2002), historical and political-economic determinants of power relations that extend far beyond relationships between, say, international consultants and area in charges at the district level. In terms of interpersonal relationships at the district level, "dominant figures—landlords, merchants, government officials, and priests—stand at a crucial point between the lives of peasants and the world beyond the villages they inhabit," Sivaramakrishnan explains, drawing on the work of Eric Wolf. "These intermediaries are nodes in the webs and nets of connection" (Sivaramakrishnan 2005, 349).

Examining how supervisors exerted power at the district level provides an entrée into wider webs of power relations. Also, the everyday techniques of power that people such as WHO employees exerted at the district level are important in their own right. It is through these strategies of everyday power that employees of the Polio Eradication Initiative attempted to ensure high immunization coverage of Pakistani children—the only way to eradicate polio.

## Everyday Power

World Health Organization and UNICEF employees had no direct control over any district employees. Since decentralization, the national government too had only limited power over the district, as discussed earlier. In the absence of direct bureaucratic systems of accountability, Polio Eradication Initiative officials resorted to a number of tactics of everyday power, including propaganda, perks, surveillance, and occasional rewards for good work, to get district-level workers to work hard on polio eradication. They also constructed a parallel bureaucracy of their own employees, from whom they could demand accountability, to perform key tasks.

## *Propaganda*

WHO and UNICEF employees in Islamabad were well aware that many people at the district level doubted that polio eradication would ever be achieved. They believed (correctly, in my view) that this affected the quality of work being performed. So they continually provided district-level workers with optimistic statements aimed at convincing people that polio eradication was imminent if work was done well.[22] For example, a bulletin sent to district officials highlighted the following "key messages" on the cover (emphases in original):

> *Pakistan is making progress* toward stopping polio.

> Polio in Pakistan has never been as geographically localized as it is now reinforcing *the possibility of success.*

> The fact that large areas in the country are without circulation of poliovirus including AJK (since 2000), FANA (since 1998), Islamabad (since 2003) and central & northern Punjab (for 2 years) reinforce that *strategies work.*

> *Polio eradication is possible* now more than ever before.

> We must *work together* to ensure eradication of polio from Pakistan.

Similarly, a cover letter with the tally sheets provided to immunization teams stated: "With the grace of Allah, the assistance of parents, and your work [*koshishon*], polio has practically disappeared from Pakistan [*taqrīban khatm ho gā'i he*]. If such work continues, polio will be completely eradicated very soon." The effectiveness of such messages was, by 2007, questionable. District-level workers had been hearing for five years that polio was on the verge of eradication, and they were skeptical of continuing declarations that the end of polio was immanent. But officials continued to make these claims.

Polio eradication planners in Islamabad also attempted to convince district-level workers to do good work through less direct means. For example, several TV spots shown across the country highlighted the work of exceptionally good supervisors and teams in the hope that the promotion of these role models would inspire other teams. Given team members' reasons for resistance, I believe it is unlikely that such spots had a large impact.

## Perks

In a few relatively rare cases, the Polio Eradication Initiative was able to sweeten its message with a significant perk such as a trip to Geneva for major decision makers and government officials. Such trips did sometimes prove effective. A CDC official mentioned to me the case of a high-level provincial elected official invited to Geneva for a meeting. There, polio eradication "captured his imagination," the CDC official said, and subsequently the Polio Eradication Initiative saw huge gains in that province. Such converts to polio eradication were valuable but rare.

## Surveillance

The Global Polio Eradication Initiative had to carry out two types of surveillance: of poliovirus circulation, and of government workers performing immunization. Surveillance of poliovirus circulation, an enormous job, involved a network of WHO employees in every area of Pakistan continuously searching for paralyzed children through visits to hospitals, clinics, and doctors.[23] When people in polio eradication talked about "surveillance," they were using the term in the public health sense, referring to surveillance of circulating poliovirus.

In addition, although it was rarely acknowledged publicly, polio eradication planners were surveilling government workers. My activities described in the last chapter are an example of this type of surveillance. Key to its success was the procurement of independent observers who would report accurately on what was happening in a given district without being drawn into local politics or local systems of patron-client relations. Polio Eradication Initiative management attempted to procure independent observers in at least two ways: by deploying international consultants, and by moving WHO employees around to different parts of the country as campaign observers.

More than forty international consultants were working on polio eradication in Pakistan, the highest concentration of such workers in any country at any time in the Polio Eradication Initiative.[24] Each international consultant cost WHO approximately $10,000 per month and taken together, their salaries, per diem, and benefits amounted to $4.5 million per year, significantly more than the combined salaries of WHO's two hundred Pakistani employees. While the amount paid international consultants was not common knowledge, most Pakistanis working on polio eradication, whether for WHO or for the government, knew it was exorbitant. Stories circulated, for example, of an international consultant living in one of Pakistan's most posh hotels.

When I began my fieldwork, this expenditure on foreigners seemed counterproductive and seemed to reflect two troubling institutional assumptions: first, that local knowledge was unimportant, and second, that Pakistanis were not capable of running an immunization program. Few international consultants spoke Urdu, much less the local languages used where they worked; they were shifted around so frequently that they never got to know much about a given district; and their high salaries, personal Land Cruisers (with drivers), and frequent travel alienated them from local culture. Officially, international consultants were in districts to provide technical support, and they were largely well credentialed, but supervising the placing of drops of vaccine in children's mouths was not an activity for which a medical specialization provided much help.

International consultants are a mainstay of many development projects, and observers have commented on precisely these issues of distance from host cultures (Jenney and Simmons 1954; Justice 1986; Pfeiffer 2004; Tendler 1975). Some have pulled no punches: Graham Hancock described international aid workers as "lords of poverty," money-hungry, arrogant bureaucrats who do not care about the needs of the poor (Hancock 1989). While I was unprepared to cast such aspersions on their character—most foreign consultants, like Dr. Ibrahim, were committed to the eradication of polio, and Pakistan was not an easy post even at such high pay—I expected to condemn foreign consultants as ineffective and expensive, much better replaced by the legions of Pakistani nationals who could be hired for the amount of one foreigner's pay.

But there is a method to the madness. Over a year in Pakistan, I came to appreciate that foreign consultants were indispensable tools to Polio Eradication Initiative planners. They were so useful for precisely what makes them unattractive to anthropologists: their alienation from Pakistani society as a whole and from their Pakistani government counterparts in particular. This separation from local culture, politics, and social relations allowed them to report honestly on what they saw, to avoid the webs of patron-clientism and politics that at times trapped even the most intelligent and scrupulous Pakistanis working at the district level, and to realistically believe that the quality of work in districts where they were posted, not their political savvy, was more likely to affect their career advancement.

In fact, Polio Eradication Initiative planners consciously worked to ensure that international consultants would retain their outsider position, mainly by reassigning them to new districts every few months. While planners valued cultural awareness—at a meeting in Geneva, some international consultants were praised for being "good at reaching out to the local community"—ultimately it was foreigners' status as outside observers that made them valuable. A high-level official in Geneva told me that "lots of internationals in a broken situation increase your span of control," and that it was the "element of outside eyes" that made them so useful; Pakistani national staff "live there," he noted, so it was "impossible" for them to get outside the system. He added, however, that in some places Pakistani national staff were more effective than international staff. "Got to have a mixture," he said. National employees were valuable for their local knowledge; international employees were, in a sense, valuable for their freedom from it.

In addition to employing foreign consultants, polio eradication planners surveilled government employees by deploying staff from one area of the country to work on campaigns in other areas. In one particularly intractable city, the dates of the campaign were shifted to get as many national and international staff as possible on hand after completing the campaign in their own districts. Similarly, the offices in Islamabad emptied out on campaign weeks, as all the WHO and UNICEF employees, national and international, traveled to different areas of the country to "support" the campaign.[25]

Planners were under the impression that such surveillance improved campaign quality. A report on an international conference call in 2003 stated that the participants agreed that "international consultants have been most effective tool in improving campaign quality" in Pakistan. Similarly, a WHO report for a public health audience on polio eradication in Pakistan stated that shifting employees to different areas during campaigns was a strategy designed "to achieve optimal coverage in areas of highest risk" (World Health Organization 2006g, 244). But with the data currently available, whether adding monitors leads to better campaigns cannot be proved. More accurate monitoring could result in lower coverage numbers for a given district, even in the context of a better campaign. However, I suspect that surveillance by outsiders does improve campaign quality.

Once while I was working on a campaign (not in Kaifabad), I stayed with my good friend Farzhana. One evening, we visited a friend of hers, Reema, for tea. There was not enough space in Reema's minuscule two rooms for her own two preschoolers, much less the four additional ones that belonged to Farzhana and me, but Reema did her best to make room for us, moving boxes of medicines outside so we would have a place to sit. (Reema's husband worked for the Health Department, Farzhana explained later, and pilfered medicine for resale to supplement his small income.)

A few days later, Farzhana told me that she had run into Reema at the corner store and asked how she was. Reema said things were hectic at her husband's work; he was an area in charge for the polio campaign. "Polio campaigns used to be relaxed," she complained, "but this time some team has come from Islamabad with some madam for checking, and everybody is scrambling. My husband had to drive over an hour in the pouring rain on his motorcycle to deliver vaccine. Even his zonal supervisor, who never shows up during the campaigns, is working hard."

Farzhana laughed and asked if Reema knew who the madam was.

Upon learning that the madam had recently been at her house for tea, Reema was annoyed. "If I'd known it was only her," she said, "I never would have let my husband drive that far in the rain at night."

In areas where outside monitors were not able to go, campaign quality was often poor. The prime example is what people in polio eradication called "security compromised areas," which were often prime locations for virus circulation. Violence and unrest were common in parts of the country—primarily the Federally Administered Tribal Areas and parts of the North-West Frontier Province bordering Afghanistan; these same areas harbored polio transmission, but not apparently as a direct result of unrest—there were nearly always windows of opportunity in which to go door-to-door.[26] Rather, all UN employees—nationals and internationals—were banned from such areas.[27] Without UN supervision, the quality of the campaigns in these areas was, in the words of one report, a "question mark." Ongoing poliovirus circulation in many of these areas indicated that campaign quality was in fact poor. While in general these districts faced a number of challenges, the continued presence of the poliovirus there suggests that "external monitors" in other areas did have a positive effect.[28]

Ultimately, however, the outside observers had no direct power. Their observations could result in public shaming and negative reports to supervisors, and their presence probably spurred people to work harder in many cases. However—and ongoing virus circulation in Pakistan is proof of this—simple surveillance without teeth in terms direct lines of accountability was not enough to ensure campaigns of the very highest quality.

### Positive Reinforcement

Aware that workers felt they were not being appreciated for doing good work, UN officials in Islamabad planned and implemented a Polio Heroes award system to recognize the best teams and area in charges. This system had not yet been fully implemented by the time I left Pakistan, so I cannot comment reliably on its effectiveness. A system recognizing good work was certainly a positive step. However, the rewards—a certificate and perhaps meeting an elected official—were purely symbolic. The system was unlikely to cause a revolution in worker motivation.

### Building Parallel Bureaucracies

Unable to exert direct control over government workers, WHO and UNICEF constructed parallel bureaucracies of their own, with workers in every district. For example, most districts had a government employee, a doctor, who was responsible for disease surveillance. However, WHO could not rely on them to search for paralyzed children, both because, as a senior WHO official explained, they often lacked "necessary enabling factors" like vehicles and fuel allowances and because, as doctors, many felt they were "too senior for fieldwork." So WHO had its own surveillance officers in every district who were in fact responsible for poliovirus surveillance in Pakistan. Initially, it had been hoped that the WHO surveillance officers would be phased out, but that never proved possible. While some government surveillance officers did work hard, the WHO surveillance officers did most of the work of visiting hospitals and doctors, searching for paralyzed children, and collecting stool samples. Because virus surveillance required only a relatively limited workforce, WHO was able to run its system almost entirely through its own employees (all Pakistani), which made the poliovirus surveillance system in Pakistan very good.

Campaigns, however, required a workforce much too large for WHO or UNICEF to create on its own; there were about 200,000 team members in Pakistan. For campaigns, they had to rely on government workers. Even so, they did their best to create a supplemental parallel system. International consultants were part of that system, as were Pakistani WHO officers at the district level like Dr. Ahmed. In addition, WHO gave about seventeen-dollar per diems during campaigns to campaign support persons, considered short-term WHO employees. WHO hired the campaign support persons and other, longer-term employees away from the government health system for a limited time. While they were working for WHO, they received substantially higher salaries than their government jobs paid; when their contracts were up, they went back to their government posts. This exercise in "capacity building" was intended to improve the government workforce. However, it also meant that many Pakistani WHO employees had deep ties to the government health system and could not operate independently of it.

The everyday techniques of power WHO and UNICEF used in Pakistan were effective; they ensured that polio eradication was the most far-reaching public health project ever carried out in that country, reaching families who had never been touched by any other health project again and again by vaccinators carrying polio drops to their doors. What the Polio Eradication Initiative achieved was nothing short of miraculous.

But it was not enough. The resistance of district-level workers was effective too, enough to prevent campaigns from being quite good enough to eradicate polio. And so, ironically, government workers in the districts were stuck with an ever-more-demanding schedule of polio campaigns.

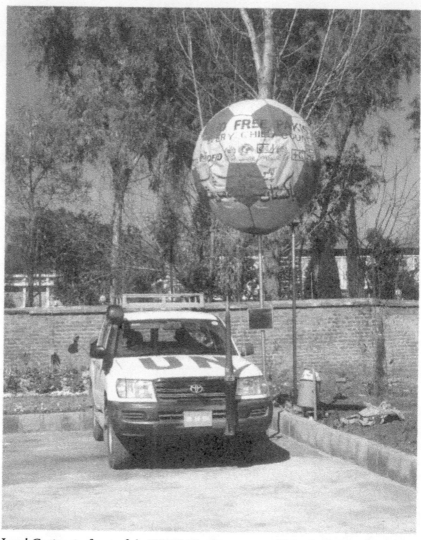

Land Cruiser in front of the WHO Headquarters in Islamabad. The plaque below the soccer ball reads, "United to Beat Polio: The Collective Final Push to Stop the Ball".... in 2003. Photo by author.

## Land Cruisers

Ahmad is a driver for the World Health Organization office in Islamabad, and Tanveer befriended him as they were both waiting in the parking lot one day. The WHO office has a huge fleet of white Toyota Land Cruisers and Hilux pickup trucks (twins of U.S. Tacomas), all of them operated by drivers. Whenever anyone working for the World Health Organization goes anywhere for work, they are required by UN security regulations to ride in one of these radio-equipped, four-wheel-drive vehicles.

The Land Cruisers are a highly visible sign of polio eradication; at one meeting I attended in a small Peshawar hotel, the large white vehicles overflowed the parking lot and blocked the road. The vehicles are a luxurious perk for the Pakistani and international employees of WHO; while high-level Pakistani government employees travel in jeeps, low-level government supervisors in the Polio Eradication Initiative use motorcycles or bicycles—often provided for the purpose with international money.

The Land Cruisers are also, at times, a real nuisance. They are useful in rural areas with bad roads but useless in Pakistan's dense city centers, much too wide to drive down the narrow alleyways of the cities and often difficult to park within walking distance of where a WHO employee needs to go. And while there is an enormous fleet of them, at the height of a vaccination campaign they can be in short supply. Some WHO employees argued with UN security staff without success that they should be able to travel without the Land Cruisers.

Ahmad has worked as a driver at WHO for several years. A driver's official job is to drive WHO employees wherever they need to go and wait for them until they are finished. In many cases this extends as far as picking them up at home and bringing them to the office each morning. Drivers also fill many additional roles on an unofficial, ad hoc basis: they are tour guides, translators, and passers-on of gossip and information obtained from drivers of Pakistani government vehicles. Ahmad's pay is around 15,000 rupees ($250) a month. This is, in general, decent pay, about 50 percent more than government drivers earn. But Ahmad is annoyed that drivers for UNICEF make nearly twice his salary. (UNICEF salaries are high for all positions, which rankles many Pakistani WHO employees, even those who by their own admission are paid decent salaries.) Moreover, like nearly everyone else working on polio eradication—in theory a temporary program—Ahmad's contract extends for only three months. Thus far, it had been renewed, but, he told Tanveer, "one month I am happy, the next I begin to worry, and the third I feel sick."

# CHAPTER 5

# Islamabad

The commitment of the government has been absolute.
—WHO international official, Technical
Advisory Group meeting, April 2007

Let me also reinforce that from the government we have
tremendous political leadership and commitment. . . .
The PM and the First Lady have been leading polio
campaigns. . . . The political leadership is absolutely clear.
—Pakistani minister of health, Technical
Advisory Group meeting, April 2007

The problem is that it's supposed to be a government
program, but it's not.
—WHO official, Islamabad

POLIO ERADICATION IN PAKISTAN was officially a government
program with support from international organizations like WHO. In certain times and places, this was how things actually worked. Since hundreds
of thousands of Pakistani government employees did the work of vaccinating children, polio eradication was a government program in a very real
sense. As one WHO official noted, the progress made in greatly reducing the number of polio cases in Pakistan would never have been possible
without government involvement.

But in another sense, polio eradication was not a Pakistani government
program; it was initiated, funded, and administered by international UN
agencies and the governments of wealthy countries like the United States,
the United Kingdom, and Japan. Pakistan took on polio eradication in
response to international directives, not because it was an issue of national
importance. For an eradication program, this internationally mandated
approach was unavoidable; if polio is to disappear entirely, every country

must simultaneously implement the recommendations of the Global Polio Eradication Initiative.[1] Still, the official line was that polio eradication was a project of the government of Pakistan.

The frequent repetition of the ideal—"polio eradication is a government program"—is an indicator of the fiction's fragility. There was an ongoing, low-level struggle in Islamabad that centered around who should be responsible for administering polio eradication. In practice, UN agencies ran the project at the national level in Islamabad. They did so in large part reluctantly, as their attempts to get government employees to take on planning and administrative duties met with significant resistance.

And yet, even as they hired large Islamabad- and field-based staffs to do the work that the Pakistani health system did not, UN agencies worked hard at maintaining the fiction of government ownership. The PowerPoints, reports, and letters that UN employees prepared were often printed on government letterhead and signed by the same government officials who represented the program at international meetings, though they usually had to be briefed beforehand by UN employees. UN employees resented this work:

> UN employee 1: The problem is ownership of the government—they are thinking that *they* are supporting *us*—
> UN employee 2: I just got call from [a government official] to put together a presentation on polio and write a speech for the minister. Well, whose program is it?
> UN employee 1: That's how it runs.

This gap between the ideal model according to UN officials and what people say actually happened is not unique to the Polio Eradication Initiative in Pakistan. On the contrary, it is a characteristic of almost all human societies. As a classic anthropology text notes:

> Two different levels of thinking may be broadly distinguished. First, there are people's notions about what they actually do, the manner in which they conceive their own social system and the world they live in. And secondly, there are their beliefs about what they and other people *ought* to do, their legal and moral values or norms. . . . Since no mortals (so far as we know) suppose themselves to inhabit the best of all possible worlds, there are always some social relationships in which real and ideal, what is and what ought to be, are distinguished. Not *all* husbands, wives, neighbours, rulers, are perfect. (Beattie 1964,.37)

Some societies have ideals driven by religious doctrine; the Polio Eradication Initiative has ideals driven by the WHO's official policy. These extremely powerful ideals drive practice in important ways, but to equate them with practice would be a mistake. In societies with ideals of honesty, fidelity, and respect for private property, people still lie, cheat, and steal (though they may be punished for it). In societies with an ideal that national governments embrace international mandates, government officials drag their feet (not, as it turns out, a punishable offense—though some UN officials probably wish it were).

## Structural Power

To grasp who creates the ideal, and why, and why it is not uniformly embraced—we must revisit the issue of power. In the previous chapter, I described several everyday techniques of power that UN employees used in attempts to cut through the resistance of low-level employees and to ensure high-quality immunization campaigns. These included, among others, the creation of propaganda, the surveillance of low-level workers, and the provision of perks and other rewards. While these everyday techniques of power are important, to limit our exploration of power relations to the observable human interactions I have thus far depicted in vignettes and concrete examples would be to miss some crucial dynamics in the Polio Eradication Initiative.

Much of the power exerted in polio eradication is what several theorists have called "structural power." Drawing on Foucault, Eric Wolf explains that "structural power shapes the social field of action so as to render some kinds of behavior possible, while making others less possible or impossible" (Wolf 1990, 587). The exertion of structural power may often be invisible; as it simply prevents certain courses of action from ever being feasible, someone observing the situation might see no conflict.[2]

As Stanley Barrett elaborates, structural power is a result of "the shape of the institutional framework of society" (Barrett 2002, 20). This framework is a global one. Paul Farmer refers to "historically given (and often economically driven) processes and forces that conspire to constrain individual agency" (Farmer 1996, 23).[3] The economic and political legacies of colonialism, for example, place government officials in charge of directing policy for the Pakistani health system in a weak position vis-à-vis international agencies and nations like the United States. When it comes time to decide what Pakistan's public health priorities are, Pakistani officials may have to defer to the desires of officials from the United States or the UN. And they may find it in their best interests to do so without argument.

Since structural power is exerted without readily apparent conflict, it can be difficult to pin down. As James C. Scott argues, the official story of those in power—what he calls the "public transcript"—is nearly always repeated aloud and in public by their subordinates, so if one sees only such public interaction, one might not be aware that there is any conflict at all. Subordinates appear, based on their own statements, to be willing supporters of the status quo. In private, however, subordinates may speak differently, and they may in fact resist the very demands that they publicly support (Scott 1990).

One way, then, to diagnose the existence of structural power is to find instances in which what people publicly agree to—the public transcript—differs from what they say in private or from what they actively support in practice. Another way to locate structural power is to find instances where public speech adheres to the official line so universally—despite compelling reasons to disagree with it—that we can reasonably infer contextual forces at work. For example, every single nation in the World Health Assembly, the World Health Organization's governing body, has expressed support for the Polio Eradication Initiative. The Initiative began with a unanimous vote of the Assembly in 1988, and in 1999, when it was clear that 2000 as the target date of eradication was unattainable, the Assembly unanimously voted to intensify the project. While there are plenty of compelling reasons to support polio eradication, there are also a number of reasons not to: it is incredibly expensive, diverts time and energy from other goals, and might not be achievable. Wealthy countries have good reason to support the goal of polio eradication because, as we will see, they will save money if it succeeds. Poor countries that have to do the work of implementing campaigns may either find the arguments for eradication compelling or feel that the risky venture is not worth the time and energy it demands. Both perspectives are reasonable, and all else being equal, one would expect at least some countries to vote against attempting the eradication of polio.

But not a single one did. The public transcript—that polio eradication was a goal worthy of significant investment and an unprecedented coordinated mobilization of people across the world in pursuit of a single health goal—went unchallenged.

The impressive size and reach of the Polio Eradication Initiative is in many ways a testament to the structural power of the United States. It is not purely a project of the United States. The polio elimination project in the Americas that became the model for the Global Polio Eradication

Initiative was certainly not reducible to a U.S. directive. However, it was possible in large part because of the support of U.S. members of Rotary, the CDC, and USAID.

Similarly, the support of the U.S. government and of U.S. members of Rotary has been critical to the Global Polio Eradication Initiative. As Peter Evans of the WHO's Expanded Programme on Immunization explained in 1994, the United States pushed hard for polio eradication in the early years of the Initiative, perhaps at the expense of other programs: "EPI [the Expanded Programme on Immunization] has been influenced by our donors. . . . [The] USA wants polio immunization. Europeans want infrastructure building [primary care]. Their fight is very big and important. . . . Expense of eradication is very high. It will take half of EPI funds" (quoted in Muraskin 1998, 72). The U.S. government, through the CDC and USAID, is the single largest donor to polio eradication, having contributed over $1 billion as of January 2008 (World Health Organization 2008b, 8).

During my research, when other major bilateral donors were becoming skeptical that eradication would be achieved, the United States had not wavered in its stated commitment to polio eradication. In interviews, representatives of several other bilateral donor organizations in Pakistan told me that they were reevaluating their contributions to polio eradication; one had reduced funding for the program. USAID showed no signs of taking such steps.

There are several major reasons for the U.S. government's support for polio eradication. Polio, unlike, say, malaria or tuberculosis, is a disease with emotional weight for many Americans, who remember outbreaks of polio in the early and mid-1900s and, with the advent of the Salk and Sabin vaccines, its eventual elimination from the United States. The U.S. membership of Rotary, which numbers nearly half a million, is no exception, and Rotary has been an effective lobby in the U.S. Congress. Bill Foege, the former director of the CDC, a veteran of the Smallpox Eradication Program, and a supporter of eradication, testified before a Senate subcommittee:

> Some people in this room will recall that April day in 1955 when a press conference at the University of Michigan announced that the Salk vaccine actually protected children against polio. It is almost impossible to recreate the feeling of that day, but the next day around the United States, simultaneously and spontaneously, there were signs in store windows that said, thank you, Dr. Salk. Well, as you know, we struggled with the best mechanisms, but we finally got it right, and 25

years after the vaccine was introduced, we had the last outbreak in this country. But we did not automatically go the next step and commit to global eradication. It took a catalyst, and as we have heard repeatedly this morning, that catalyst was Rotary International. It was not just the resources that we have heard about of millions of hours of work or millions of dollars. It was their role as a collective conscience. Gandhi once said that his interpretation of the Golden Rule is that he should not be able to enjoy something denied to others, and Rotary reminded us that we cannot enjoy having our children and grandchildren free from polio unless we give all parents that same joy. (U.S. Congress 1999, 31)

In addition to the moral imperative invoked by Foege, the United States has financial reasons to support polio eradication. Its achievement would mean that, ultimately, polio immunization in the United States could be halted.[4] In the 1990s, the United States spent on the order of $250 million a year for oral polio vaccine (Taylor, Cutts, and Taylor 1997).[5] Achievement of polio eradication could result in significant financial savings for the United States.

In light of such economic benefits, the question arises of whether the Polio Eradication Initiative serves mainly the poor countries carrying out immunization activities—or the rich countries financing them. In a place like Pakistan, the burden of disease due to polio is minor compared to other health conditions.[6] If polio eradication activities draw resources away from diseases with a much higher burden of morbidity and mortality, the net effect of the program could be negative.

Therefore, it is a topic of lively and ongoing debate whether polio eradication activities contribute to or detract from routine immunization and from primary health care more generally. A number of studies report the effects of the Polio Eradication Initiative on health systems more generally (Bonu, Rani, and Baker 2003; Bonu, Rani, and Razum 2004; Levin, Ram, and Kaddar 2002; Loevinsohn et al. 2002; Pan American Health Organization 1995). The equivocal results of most of these studies spring from the same major problem: since mass polio vaccination has been carried out in every poor country in the world, no comparison cases exist of countries that were *not* involved in the Polio Eradication Initiative. Also, in many countries major health system reforms, like decentralization in Pakistan, took place around the same time mass vaccination activities were scaled up. As one major study notes: "Relatively little is known about the opportunity costs of polio eradication" (Loevinsohn et al. 2002, 19).

In 1995, after polio elimination had been achieved in the Americas, a Pan American Health Organization study on this issue concluded: "Overall, the Expanded Program on Immunization/Polio had a positive effect on health systems in the Americas. However, the findings of this commission should be understood in the perspective of the reality that most countries in the Americas already had a well organized health system and infrastructure when Polio/EPI was started" (Pan American Health Organization 1995, 8). Polio Eradication Initiative employees cited this report as evidence that mass vaccination activities have positive "spillover" effects (e.g., Aylward, Hull, et al. 2000; Sutter and Cochi 1997).

However, several of the report's authors published an article in which they argued that since polio eradication's primary financial benefit will accrue to wealthy countries, and since polio's effects on overall morbidity and mortality are minor compared to those of other major diseases, it is "shortsighted for donors to use their considerable influence to promote polio eradication if this delays or diverts long-term investment by poor countries in sustainable health systems." Further, "the benefits of polio eradication in the Americas can be directly applied to policy-making only in countries with established and sustainable health systems, strong leadership and central and district levels, a well-organized infrastructure, and local ownership and decision making." Drawing on a report addressing experiences in Africa (UNICEF 1996), they pointed out that the experiences of resource-poor countries without strong infrastructure were often not so positive. Polio eradication would be an ethical goal, they argued, only if rich countries used the money they saved by stopping vaccination in their own countries to build broader public health infrastructure in poor countries (Taylor, Cutts, and Taylor 1997, 924).

Polio Eradication Initiative officials responded by asserting that it was poor countries themselves who had signed on to polio eradication activities, that heads of state had endorsed polio eradication at international conferences, and that government health departments were themselves carrying out mass vaccination campaigns (Lee et al. 1998). "We appreciate that the authors have made known their concerns," several CDC officials wrote, "and welcome the opportunity to report that developing countries are capable of making their own rational health decisions" (Sutter and Cochi 1997). But given the structural power of the major backers of the Polio Eradication Initiative, poor countries had little choice but to give the project at least lip service.

District-level government health department employees in Pakistan largely felt that polio vaccination campaigns detracted from other activities, and I suspect they are correct. However, while I certainly do not defend polio eradication unequivocally, its significant achievements should not be overlooked. The considerable resources and single-minded focus of the Polio Eradication Initiative in Pakistan resulted in the vaccination (although only for one disease) of populations previously almost beyond the reach of government health services. Other achievements of the Polio Eradication Initiative, such as the creation of a sensitive and comprehensive disease surveillance system in Pakistan (albeit one staffed entirely by WHO), have the potential to improve prevention of other infectious diseases in the future. Whether such infrastructure will continue to be funded once the Polio Eradication Initiative ends remains to be seen.

Whether the net effects of the Polio Eradication Initiative on health in Pakistan were positive or negative, however, its existence was a manifestation of the structural power of countries like the United States. Polio eradication is not a U.S. program; the U.S. government's contributions, while substantial, cover only around a fifth of the total cost of the project, and administering a program simultaneously in every country of the world would have been impossible without the involvement of an organization like WHO. But U.S. enthusiasm for polio eradication carried much more weight in world policy making than did the lack of enthusiasm of a government of a place like Pakistan.

Pakistani government officials never publicly voiced ambivalence about the program—as this chapter's epigraphs attest, they were publicly supportive. But national government officials did resist polio eradication's mandates. A program of mass vaccination for measles in Pakistan that began during my time there provides an excellent example of the process by which structural power can silence opposition.

## Measles Elimination:
## The Unwanted Project Everyone Agreed To

In early 2007, as polio cases continued to appear in several areas of Pakistan, a new and ambitious program of measles control began its pilot phases in that country. The project, which initially aimed to reduce the incidence of measles by 50 percent, was part of the Measles Initiative, a program modeled on the Global Polio Eradication Initiative. The WHO's Eastern Mediterranean Region had set a goal of eliminating measles in its region by 2010. Achieving this goal (widely viewed as unrealistic—the product, one WHO official told me, of a "global competition" for goals among WHO regions) would require a number of mass measles-immunization campaigns in Pakistan. As Pakistan had a large population with a high rate of measles, lowering the measles count there was becoming an international priority.[7]

The organization of measles immunization campaigns and the creation of a measles surveillance system in Pakistan were huge jobs. But the Measles Initiative had dedicated only one UN employee to the country; after all, it was a government program. While the hiring of additional staff was planned, they had not yet materialized as of 2007. The WHO polio eradication staff, already working sixty-hour weeks, were now expected to take on the planning, implementation, and surveillance of campaigns for yet another disease. Government employees were to be responsible for yet more campaigns on top of polio campaigns, giving them even less time to deal with other health issues. Measles vaccine, unlike the polio vaccine used in Pakistan, was injectable rather than oral and thus required trained workers to give shots; also unlike polio vaccine, it could have serious side effects if administered incorrectly.

It is not surprising, then, that neither government employees nor WHO employees were enthusiastic about the Measles Initiative. The mystery to many was why the Pakistani government had agreed to take on measles campaigns at all.

"I don't know why," one foreign representative of a bilateral aid agency told me. "Maybe they cannot say no."

A polio eradication official in Geneva had an answer. "It was really pushed on the Ministry of Health by WHO and UNICEF."

The structural power of the major partners in the Measles Initiative—including the CDC, the Red Cross, WHO, and UNICEF—was sufficient to ensure implementation of a major new health initiative in Pakistan even when the timing seemed bad to everyone involved. The feeling of many in Pakistan—government officials as well as Pakistani and international WHO officials—that it would be better to implement measles campaigns only when the burden of polio campaigns was lighter was not sufficient to counter the structural power of the Measles Initiative's major international partners and donors.[8]

A stream of foreign consultants visited Islamabad to assist with getting the Measles Initiative off the ground; they were largely, probably justifiably, upset about the lack of progress toward implementing campaigns in Pakistan. At one meeting, a particularly frustrated CDC official repeatedly asked a government official: "Does the minister know there's a measles campaign?" (The government official remained sullenly silent in response to these questions.) "Be sure to tell the minister there's a measles campaign," the CDC official continued, ostensibly as a joke, but nobody laughed. He instructed the government official to collect additional information from districts and to implement an information campaign for doctors in Pakistan, who were apparently largely unaware that measles vaccination campaigns were about to begin.

After the meeting, the government official, who had remained largely silent during the formal meeting, complained to a Pakistani WHO employee in Urdu:

> They should deal with these things themselves. They have 110 kinds of meetings—meetings upon meetings. And they have unrealistic expectations—you need three weeks for the stuff they want immediately. As for the complaints about doctors not knowing about the campaign, whose responsibility was that? And why didn't they collect data themselves at district meetings? Now they want me to collect data from all of the districts. I swear to God, I'm upset by their style of demanding things.

This government official, who was supposed to be running the program, found himself treated like an underling of foreign officials. It rankled.

Also clear in the government official's frustrated outburst was that, despite the official line, he did not consider measles control to be a Pakistani government program. Rather, since it was the international organizations that had insisted on measles campaigns being initiated, he felt they should take responsibility for carrying out the work of the campaigns. "They should deal with these things themselves," he said, indicating that he felt measles control was not his purview. "Whose responsibility was that?" he asked rhetorically.

In fact, on paper, nearly all Measles Initiative activities were the responsibility of the government. The lone UNICEF official responsible for supporting measles vaccination in Pakistan attempted to get government officials to carry out training, planning, and pilot campaigns. But given the attitudes of these officials to the project, it is not surprising that implementation of measles campaigns was hopelessly behind schedule.

It is significant—and diagnostic of structural power—that while there was widespread discussion in private at all levels of the Polio Eradication Initiative about dissatisfaction with concurrent implementation of measles campaigns, such sentiments were rarely aired publicly. The government official just quoted aired his dissatisfaction in Urdu after the meeting; during the meeting, when international officials could understand him, he had not voiced such complaints in English. If one were to rely on official statements, one would see only a positive synergy between polio and measles campaigns. The Polio Eradication Initiative's literature states that, as part of "mainstreaming" polio eradication, a goal is for all countries to have "polio operations . . . fully integrated with those for measles" (World Health Organization 2004).[9] Similarly, a weekly surveillance update e-mail from the WHO Pakistan office in November 2007 stated:

> Supplementary immunization activities for measles are currently be-ing conducted in Sindh province and the remaining uncovered areas of NWFP and Balochistan. Polio eradication staff is supporting the moni-toring of these activities. In high risk populations, especially in areas where there is difficult access to all children, oral polio vaccine (OPV) is also being given. Anecdotal feedback from the field shows that there is great acceptance for measles vaccination from the community. Many refusals have been covered during the measles campaign in areas like South & North Waziristan Agencies.

Here it is suggested that implementation of measles campaigns has made certain populations more accepting of polio vaccine.[10] Many polio plan-ners were concerned about the opposite effect—that the implementation of measles campaigns on top of polio campaigns would leave health work-ers and parents tired of immunization drives and less likely to immunize children against polio. That there were areas in which measles campaigns did in fact assist with polio eradication activities is doubtless true. How-ever, only the positive effects of measles campaigns were aired publicly. That the negative effects were discussed only in private is an indication of structural power in operation (see Scott 1990). This positive spin also reflects the strength of the culture of optimism in the World Health Organization.

## Resistance in Islamabad

There was no such visible conflict in Islamabad over the use of mass po-lio campaigns as a public health strategy in Pakistan—likely because they had been around so long that the issue had largely already been decided. (Door-to-door campaigns in Pakistan started in 1999, about eight years before I began my research.) Perhaps as a result of this long experience, polio eradication officials—unlike measles planners—had long ago given up on getting government officials to do routine activities for them. At one meeting, there was a discussion of getting the Ministry of Health to send a letter to a district with some problems in the surveillance system. A high-level Pakistani WHO official argued successfully that rather than get the government to send a letter, the WHO should send it themselves. If left to the government, "it will get stuck in the bureaucratic chain," he said, shrugging his shoulders.

Polio eradication staff held twice-weekly planning meetings in a government office for officials from WHO, UNICEF, and the government. "We are trying to convince our governmental colleagues that this is their meeting," a WHO official explained; "otherwise our conference room is much more comfortable." However, government officials were often not present. "Same people here, same people missing, same excuses," another WHO official sighed one day.

When WHO officials did try to get high-level government officials to perform tasks for polio eradication, they often met with resistance. Take, for instance, the following exchange following a request from a WHO official that high-level government officials visit poor-performing districts where WHO officials could not go because of security restrictions:

> Government official 1: The provincial government can take the lead on it.
> Government official 2: We can write a letter or can arrange a meeting—how many districts are there?
> WHO official: Six or seven.
> Government official 2: They will be happy to come here.
> WHO official: It's better if you go to the province . . .
> Government official 1: The provincial office should take the lead.
> Government official 2: We can write a letter.
> WHO official: My suggestion is this—if we want zero transmission by May, now is the time—a high-level federal-level mission going from Islamabad to this area.
> Government official 2: When?
> WHO official: Within a week's time.
> Government official 2: Dr. A's availability is very important and Dr. A is not available next week.

In this exchange, the request that high-level government officials go to a key area of poliovirus transmission was deflected with arguments that oversight was the province's responsibility, that people from the areas in question "would be happy" to come to Islamabad, and that key officials were "not available."

In February of 2007, two Pakistani health employees working on polio immunization activities were killed and a third injured by a car bomb in

Bajour, in Pakistan's Tribal Areas. Government and WHO officials agreed that a government award and monetary support for the families of these workers were important gestures. In late February, government officials said that they planned to recognize the men with a national award, and by March 1, the CDC had sent checks of a thousand dollars for each of the three families to Islamabad. Subsequently, the government approved additional compensation for the families. High-level government officials were supposed to travel to the area to deliver the checks and present the national award—but they never did. The issue came up repeatedly in meetings over the following months.

*March 22*
Government official: The minister of health will be in Nowshera on the eighth; we can visit the family and hand over the check then.
WHO official: Make sure the check is ready.
Government official: The secretary [of health] had very kindly agreed to present the family with a civil award, we just need to decide which one.
WHO official: Great, that's very good.

*April 5*
WHO official: The government funds have still not arrived. . . . The minister of health's planned trip to Nowshera was a very good plan but [smiling] unfortunately it did not materialize.

*April 12*
Government official 1: The checks are ready, but we are just waiting how we will deliver these checks.
Government official 2: We did plan a visit by the minister but . . .
Government official 1: During the NIDs [polio campaign] we can plan to take him.
Government official 3: Civil awards would not be a bad idea.
Government official 2: The previous secretary of health agreed to civil awards but . . .

*May 14*
UNICEF official: Dr. B [the government official quoted on March 22] said they should come here to Islamabad to get the checks. He said [imitating his voice], "A thousand dollars is nothing—why a big ceremony for that?"

WHO official: It is becoming embarrassing.
UNICEF official: Just give them the money so they can use it.

*May 17*
Government official: The minister was supposed to go but he didn't.
I absolutely agree with you—it's more respectful to do the ceremony in Nowshera than to make the families come to Islamabad. It
should be done as soon as possible.

The checks were ultimately given to the families in Islamabad in early
June, three months after the CDC checks had arrived.

Verbal agreement from government officials on the importance of
traveling to the area to present civil awards was forthcoming—but action
was not. Such foot-dragging and false compliance were government officials' primary modes of everyday resistance in Islamabad. As in the case
of measles, government officials made it clear through their actions and
the occasional comment that polio eradication was really a UN program,
even if they were going along with it. WHO and UNICEF officials' arse-
nal of techniques of everyday power to overcome this resistance was quite
slim in Islamabad. They could not perform surveillance on the minister
of health; and as we will see, their propaganda had little impact on high-
level government officials. They were left with perks; the minister of health
and high-level immunization officials were regularly flown to Geneva and
Cairo for meetings. Structural power was sufficient to ensure spoken support for polio eradication but not to get government officials to make it
their first priority.

In public statements, government officials in Islamabad said they were
completely personally committed to the goal of eradication. "Polio is our
number one health strategy," said the minister of health to WHO officials
visiting from Geneva. (He did immediately diminish the strength of this
statement by saying that the "alongside number one strategy" was routine
immunization.) However, in my ten months working on polio eradication
in Pakistan, I saw the minister of health only that once. High-level government officials' support of polio eradication was impressive in speech but
lukewarm in practice.

# Decision Making and Accountability:
# The Case of Monovalent Vaccines

The extent of the structural power UN organizations and other partners like the CDC possess can be best seen in cases where government and UN officials disagree on a given issue. A case in point is the controversy over monovalent vaccines.

There are three distinct types of poliovirus, called Type 1, Type 2, and Type 3. Type 2 has apparently been eradicated; no circulating Type 2 poliovirus has been observed since 1999. Type 1 and Type 3 are still with us. Type 1 is the more virulent, causing paralysis in a higher percentage of the people it infects. Type 1 is also more likely to spread over long distances, even internationally; Type 3, as a CDC virologist observed, "stays home."

Immunity to one type of poliovirus does not confer immunity to the other two types. Thus, polio vaccines have traditionally contained all three types of poliovirus—hence called "trivalent" vaccines.

In 2005, with financial support from the Gates Foundation, the Global Polio Eradication Initiative introduced monovalent oral polio vaccines, which confer immunity to only one type of poliovirus. Their advantage is that they are better at producing immunity for the specific type of virus they target. For example, in India monovalent oral Type 1 polio vaccine (mOPV1) protects 80 percent of children against wild poliovirus Type 1 after five doses, compared to fourteen doses for trivalent vaccine (Grassly et al. 2007).[11] The disadvantage of monovalent vaccines is, of course, that they protect against only one of the two currently circulating types of poliovirus.

The official rhetoric in the international community upon the development of mOPV1 was optimistic. Monovalent vaccines were touted as a key to achieving eradication. Steve Cochi of the CDC was quoted in an official report as saying: "All the other countries eradicated poliovirus using trivalent OPV alone, while monovalent OPV types 1 and 3 are now available, providing potent, additional tools" (World Health Organization 2006c). The global Advisory Committee on Polio Eradication met in late 2005 and concluded, according to WHO reports, that "with sufficient resources and expanded use of mOPV1, all polio-affected countries except Nigeria can stop this disease by mid-2006" (World Health Organization 2006b).

There was only one case of Type 3 paralytic polio in Pakistan in 2005, and international experts concluded that Pakistan should be using monovalent Type 1 vaccine instead of the trivalent vaccine used thus far. An "informal technical consultation" held in May of 2005 concluded,

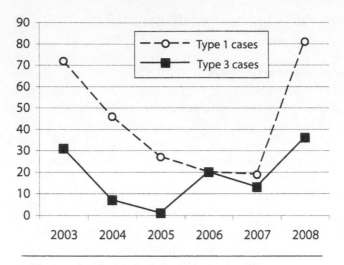

**Figure 6. Polio cases in Pakistan by type, 2003–2008**

The predominance of Type 1 poliovirus in the remaining transmission in Pakistan suggests that the programme is reaching the stage where use of monovalent OPV type 1 can provide important advantages in stopping the remaining chains of transmission; . . . the programme should plan for the use of mOPV1 in both the September 2005 NID [National Immunization Days] and the November 2005 SNID [Subnational Immunization Days] rounds. The Ministry of Health should ensure that the necessary steps for approval of use of mOPV1 in Pakistan are taken as quickly as possible. (World Health Organization 2005c)

Given the international enthusiasm for monovalent vaccines, Pakistani government officials had little choice but to license and use mOPV1; they were also, at least publicly, supportive of its adoption. The minister of health gave his spoken support to the plan both in Geneva and in Islamabad (Maqbool 2005; World Health Organization 2006h).

However, the introduction of mOPV1 in Pakistan did not have quite the effect that was hoped. By the end of 2006, forty cases of paralytic polio were found in Pakistan, up from twenty-eight in 2005 (see Figure 6). The use of mOPV1 was associated with a reduction in the number of Type 1 cases, to twenty in 2006 compared to twenty-seven in 2005. The unintended side effect of the use of mOPV1 in Pakistan, however, was a resurgence of Type 3 poliovirus in the country: twenty cases of paralytic Type 3 polio in 2006, up from only one in 2005.

With this setback, the extent to which government workers at a number of levels perceived the decision to use mOPV1 in late 2005 and early 2006 as the World Health Organization's imperative, and not a decision for which the Pakistani health system was responsible, became clear. Government employees in districts with outbreaks of Type 3 virus and officials at the national level criticized the WHO and its partner agencies for having made a bad decision. Ultimately, the issue was who was to blame for the increase in cases in 2006 over 2005: district employees and government workers for poor campaigns, or international policy makers for introducing mOPV1 too soon, before Type 3 virus had really disappeared from Pakistan. This issue surfaced at a Technical Advisory Group meeting of international policy makers in Islamabad in April of 2007. A pediatrician from Karachi asked of the use of mOPV1, "Was it premature?"

A WHO official responded that campaign quality was the important issue, "whatever type of vaccine you are using."

After some discussion of the patterns of transmission of Type 3 polio, another WHO official defended the use of the monovalent vaccine. "This vaccine has worked," he said. "We knew there were going to be risks. I still believe very much that [using mOPV1] was absolutely the right decision."

The report prepared by the Technical Advisory Group highlighted "successful introduction of mOPV1 with a subsequent clear impact on WPV1 [Type 1] transmission."

Pakistani WHO officials had already disseminated optimistic messages regarding mOPV1 in Pakistan. The surveillance bulletin sent to districts in April 2007, for example, stated in bold letters on the front page, "In 2007, for the first time ever, there are *fewer type 1 polio cases than type 3 cases* in key endemic areas suggesting that the strategy of wide-scale *use of monovalent oral polio vaccine type 1 (mOPV1)*—which protects children twice as fast against type 1 polio than the traditionally-used trivalent OPV—*is working*" (emphasis in original).

The documents that the World Health Organization prepared for an international audience were also resolutely optimistic regarding the use of mOPV1 in Pakistan. A document from the Eastern Mediterranean Region in Cairo stated, "The strategic measures adopted by the programme since 2004 . . . as well as the use of monovalent OPV type 1 (mOPV1) have led to substantial improvements in the quality of supplementary immunization activities and in the immunization status of children in Pakistan" (World Health Organization 2006f, 7). The Global Polio Eradication's annual report for 2006 stated, "In a demonstration of the impact of mOPV1, no type 1 polio cases have been reported from reservoir areas in northern Sindh since 2005 and southern Punjab since July 2006" (World Health Organization 2007a).

Members of the international Technical Advisory Group argued that monovalent Type 3 vaccine (mOPV3) was the answer to the problems caused by mOPV1. For example, when a foreign consultant (known for speaking his mind) opined that an outbreak of Type 3 polio in north Sindh was due to the use of mOPV1 in that area, a person who worked in Sindh responded, "When we get monovalent type 3 vaccine, that will be the right response for chasing the virus in that area." A high-ranking WHO official from Geneva said, "I am very satisfied with that response."

International officials from Geneva and Atlanta told Pakistani officials to license and begin use of mOPV3. When the minister of health came to the Technical Advisory Group meeting, a high-ranking WHO official requested that mOPV3 be licensed for use in Pakistan as soon as possible. "It is a bold thing to throw at the feet of the minister," he said, "but this will make a difference."

Licensure of mOPV3 was purely a government responsibility, not in the hands of WHO employees in Islamabad, and it proceeded much more slowly than WHO officials would have liked. In fact, the requests by the officials at the Technical Advisory Group meeting to the minister came several months after the government was supposed to have been processing the licensing of mOPV3. In response to WHO officials' complaints about slowness as the vaccine remained unlicensed in May, one government official shrugged his shoulders. "It's not our fault," he said. "They [the vaccine manufacturer] didn't submit the paperwork." Monovalent Type 3 vaccine was licensed for use in Pakistan in June—later than WHO officials considered ideal, but earlier than many of them had dared to expect.

Decisions about the type of vaccine to use in a given area—mOPV1, mOPV3, or trivalent vaccine—are judgment calls; the monovalent vaccines were new, and international experts in Geneva and Atlanta, and WHO officials in Islamabad, did their best when deciding what vaccines to use in what area. My aim here is not to second-guess those decisions; rather, I want to point out that these decisions take place in the context of contested power relations and can engender resistance.

Officials at the WHO and the CDC decide which polio vaccines will be developed, licensed, and used. Cultural characteristics of these organizations influence the decisions, including optimism about the ease with which eradication will be achieved and belief in technological solutions to health problems (cf. Packard 1997). Officials in Geneva and Atlanta offer only recommendations or advice to national governments on these issues, but government officials, while they may resist through techniques like foot-dragging, have little choice but to follow the recommendations of international experts. International officials gave their advisory capacity substantial lip service—claiming, for example, that licensing a mono-valent vaccine was "a bold thing to throw at the feet of the minister"—but their structural power was such that the minister had little choice but to comply.

The response of the World Health Organization to strong arguments that international officials had miscalculated in the case of mOPV1 in Pakistan was an interesting one. Institutional optimism was so strong that admitting even a minor setback was not an option. Instead, a question-able decision was recast as a step forward: mOPV1 was "working," it had an "impact." If mOPV1 had *any* drawbacks, they would be solved by mOPV3. Government officials, who had little choice but to accept the recommendation that they license mOPV3, were skeptical.

Their skepticism was perhaps justified. Currently, a mix of mOPV1, mOPV3, and trivalent vaccines are used in Pakistan. Nonetheless, 2008 was the worst year for both types of polio in Pakistan in recent history (see Figure 6). Monovalent vaccines, while useful tools, are far from magic bullets.

## Optimism and Pessimism in Islamabad

Back in August of 2000, the *Lancet* reported on Pakistan's progress in po-lio eradication:

> Despite containing poliovirus transmission for the first time, Pakistan will not be able to eradicate poliomyelitis by the end of this year, the deadline set by WHO in 1998 for global eradication of polio, health officials said last week. "We will hopefully stop the spread of the virus by June next year, but it is almost impossible to eradicate it by [the end of] 2000," Mohammad Azam (National Institute of Health, Islamabad, Pakistan) told *The Lancet*. Last week, WHO Medical Officer, Anthony Mounts argued that the country could completely eradicate polio by the year 2000, but Azam disagreed. (Ahmad 2000)

In 2000, then, WHO officials argued that eradication in Pakistan was pos-sible on a very short time frame; government officials took a less optimis-tic and, in retrospect, much more realistic stance. The situation had not changed in 2005, when I did my pilot research. The WHO medical officer was confident that polio would be eradicated in Pakistan by the time I began my fieldwork in late 2006; his government counterpart was confident that it would not.

I am reluctant to draw firm conclusions as to why government officials in Islamabad resisted the demands of the Polio Eradication Initiative. I never felt comfortable or close enough with any high-level government official to speak frankly about this issue. Certainly they desired the eradication of polio, though this goal was not and would never be a high priority for Musharraf's administration given the other problems facing the country. However, government officials' realism, when compared to UN optimism, provides a plausible theory.

Pakistan was not in a position to refuse to carry out a major goal of UNICEF and the World Health Organization. Compliance was requisite. Once Pakistan agreed to a major health initiative, there was, in the words of one high-level government official, "intense pressure" to meet stated goals. But these goals were often wildly optimistic, perhaps impossible in the time frame provided. That UN officials would meet with government resistance in this scenario is not entirely surprising.

Government officials were tossed on the winds of global health fads. International mandates from the Global Alliance for Vaccines and Immunizations, the Polio Eradication Initiative, and the Measles Initiative left little space for government officials to shape vaccination policy in Pakistan. This is not necessarily a bad thing—health initiatives have long been at the bottom of the Pakistani government's agenda, and the country's health indicators are unimpressive—but it does shape the way government officials approach what are ostensibly their own health projects.[12]

## Policy: The Power of an Ideal

Early in my research, I spoke with a UN official frustrated with the Pakistani government's lack of commitment to polio eradication. She spoke wistfully of Ethiopia, which had no government to speak of, where the WHO was able to step in and do what needed to be done to eradicate polio. She mentioned that if Musharraf could just get the army to conduct vaccination campaigns, that strategy would probably be more effective.[13] At the time, such sentiments were distasteful to me; they were uncomfortably neocolonial. But later, the logic of her arguments began to carry some weight. I began to wonder why WHO and UNICEF didn't carry out campaigns themselves in districts where government resistance was all but insurmountable.

I asked that question of another UN official later on in my fieldwork. "Because it's a government program," she said, "and that would just entrench the idea—" She broke off. I finished for her: "That it's actually a UN program and government ownership is a farce?" She nodded and shrugged.

The Polio Eradication Initiative needed the Pakistani government to carry out eradication campaigns in Pakistan, because no other organization had the reach, especially in security-compromised areas, to marshal the workforce of more than 200,000 people needed to immunize children during campaigns. As another WHO official pointed out, the contribution of government employee time was considerable. The Polio Eradication Initiative did not have the money or the reach to create such an extensive organization without the government's assistance. Also, the widespread perception among the Pakistani population that polio vaccination was a government initiative was important in a populace often distrustful of foreign intervention.

Still, there was no a priori reason that, in theory, UN organizations could not have used the government health system to run vaccination campaigns in most of the country and done the work themselves in the relatively limited areas where there was poor campaign quality as evidenced by ongoing virus circulation. However, as the UN official's comment indicates, the ideal of polio eradication's being a government program, regardless of how things worked in practice, prevented such blatant bypassing of the government. It also prevented UN officials from using tactics such as threats or coercion of either government employees or parents who refused vaccination for their children.

The ideal represented by policy does not determine what happens on the ground, as I mentioned at the beginning of this chapter. David Mosse has argued that in development projects, policy is not even designed to reflect what is happening in implementation. The function of policy, he argues, is to get multiple stakeholders on board and, speaking in the same terms, to frame projects for donors; it does not necessarily deeply shape how projects are implemented (Mosse 2005).

It is undoubtedly the case that polio eradication policy was shaped more powerfully by international development rhetoric and culture than by the exigencies of vaccination in Pakistani cities. But policy ideals had very real effects in the Polio Eradication Initiative. The ideal that polio eradication would be a government program in Pakistan meant that while

WHO and donor countries had the structural power to get the program put in place and to ensure that the Pakistani government vaccinated thirty million children multiple times a year, they were limited in their ability to ensure accountability for performance or to cross lines that would interfere with the appearance of government control.

It is for these reasons that WHO officials consistently lamented their inability to take action. As official after official noted, they knew what the problems were and which districts they existed in. But they could not do anything to change what was happening on the ground because of the policy directive that governments own polio eradication. UN employees in Islamabad found themselves in the unenviable position of being accountable to their superiors in Cairo and Geneva for the progress of polio eradication, responsible for planning nationwide vaccination campaigns, and yet unable to exercise any real control over the practices of vaccination in Pakistan.

## Development and the State

Much current work on the relationship between development projects and nation-states focuses on the trend in the neoliberal era for NGOs to take on many tasks formerly carried out by national governments (Ferguson 2006; Pfeiffer 2004; Sharma 2006; Sharma and Gupta 2006). James Ferguson and Akhil Gupta write of "an emerging system of transnational governmentality" characterized by "the outsourcing of the functions of the state to NGOs and other ostensibly nonstate agencies" by international agencies (Ferguson and Gupta 2002, 982). As Gupta and Aradhana Sharma explain:

> Neoliberal governmentality is characterized by a competitive market logic and a focus on smaller government that operates from a distance. Neoliberalism works by multiplying sites for regulation and domination through the creation of autonomous entities of government that are not part of the formal state apparatus and are guided by enterprise logic. This government-at-a-distance involves social institutions such as nongovernmental organizations, schools, communities, and even individuals that are not part of any centralized state apparatus and are made responsible for activities formerly carried out by state agencies. Neoliberalism thus represents a shift in the rationality of government and in the shape and nature of states. (Gupta and Sharma 2006, 277)

Many of these theorists point out that the national state is not the only entity involved in governance, and that the boundaries of the state are neither obvious nor clear (Abrams 1977; cf. Asad 2004). These points are well taken.

But these trends are not universal. The involvement of NGOs is not threatening government control over the Pakistani health sector. Outside of earthquake-affected areas, where NGOs have proliferated with such abandon that (to the chagrin of evicted tenants) they have taken over many of the buildings left standing, few NGOs are particularly visible in Pakistan.[14] UN officials in the Polio Eradication Initiative could not get around the Pakistani government even if they wanted to. No other organization was extensive enough to carry out the activities necessary for the eradication of polio. Further, UN officials were tied to the ideal of polio eradication's being a government program.

Not that taking on the task of administering polio campaigns significantly buttressed the power of the Pakistani government. It is often argued in the anthropological literature on development agencies, most famously by James Ferguson (Ferguson 1994), that administration of a development project expands the power of the entity administering it, whether that is a nation-state or an NGO. But the Polio Eradication Initiative is too narrowly focused on the administration of oral polio vaccine to have significant wide-reaching effects in *any* arena. Unlike some development projects studied by anthropologists (Ferguson 1994; Li 2007), the Initiative does not aim to remake society but only to administer oral polio vaccine. Its side effects, whether positive or negative, are, I believe, minimal.[15] The existence of the Polio Eradication Initiative was less about the expansion of state bureaucratic power than about the limits of that power, as government employees at all levels were harnessed to a task they were not enthusiastic about.

The landscape of the distribution of power between nation-states and international organizations is multilayered and complex. The shift represented by neoliberalism is far from total. Even as international organizations, both multilateral and bilateral, work around national governments in some development projects, they are tied by their own rhetoric or by practical necessity to working directly through them in others. In such cases, power struggles between international organizations and governments—conflicts, often just below the surface, over who gets to make major policy decisions and who is held accountable for reaching goals—are common, fluid, and ongoing. They are likely, in many cases, to determine the success and failure of the development projects to which both international organizations and national governments claim to be committed.

## Inequality, Resistance, and Polio Transmission

The underlying reason for the difficulties the Polio Eradication Initiative faced in Pakistan was simply that the task was so difficult. As many as ten doses of Oral Polio Vaccine are necessary to confer immunity against polio to children living in many areas of South Asia, as I have noted. In much of the country, fewer than 60 percent of children have received routine (as opposed to campaign-based) immunizations, including the basic three doses of OPV—which points to the dual challenges of poor health infrastructure and the need for even more doses of vaccine to be administered during campaigns.

The populations where poliovirus is still circulating in Pakistan are the country's most marginalized and impoverished: Afghani refugees, nomads, residents of urban slums. In my own survey of these groups in and around Kaifabad, I found polio immunization coverage low (less than 80 percent in my sample of people living in tents and temporary housing had been covered in the last round). It was not that these groups were against vaccination; they were almost universally in favor of it. The lady health workers I interviewed made similar observations. "These people are so cooperative," one commented. "There isn't a single one that is a refusal." Another told me: "As soon as they see me, they run to bring their children to me. They take more of an interest in giving their children vaccine than others do."

But a few lady health workers mentioned that they were reluctant to cover these groups. One explained:

> Look, I was scared because, one, the houses are far apart, and, two, Pathans live there. I'm scared of Pathans. They say, "Who is this, who's come here?" There were two of us, we were both women, we went there to given them polio drops. Well, in one tent there was a pregnant woman. She was in pain. She said, "Come here." We were scared, we didn't know what was inside, so I made out a referral slip and told her to go to the health post, that there was a Lady Health Visitor there that would help with her delivery. There, those Pathans' children are dirty too, bare feet, in a horrible state. There are some places I just don't want to go to give polio drops. But what to do, it's a job. I have to go.[16]

"I'm scared of their dogs," another lady health worker explained, "and on top of that they're Pathans, they don't listen." Yet another mentioned that she didn't like going into tents, so she would call all the children in such settlements together to a central point.

Several team members working in rural areas said mobile populations were inconvenient to cover because they were located far from villages covered during campaigns. As one woman told me, "They live far away, and there are these uninhabited areas, and jungle—we two ladies have to cross these areas."

And there were other issues. Beggars often took their young children with them into the streets, leaving their tents empty. Chalking and record-keeping in tent colonies were sometimes difficult, and coming back to find a missed child was often deemed not worth the trouble. Team members' resistance to the demands placed on them intensified when they were working in areas where they would rather not be.

But it is not just the neglect of lady health workers that makes these populations vulnerable to polio. Nonexistent sanitation infrastructure, overcrowded small tents or homes (sometimes constructed, of necessity, amidst the garbage dumps of wealthier home dwellers), and inadequate nutrition conspire to leave these populations prey to a number of diseases. Their marginalization makes them the most likely targets of infectious disease—and simultaneously the hardest to reach through population-level interventions. They play an important role in sustaining polio transmission.[17]

Still, as I mentioned previously, if three doses of vaccine were all that were required to confer immunity to polio in Pakistan, elimination would likely have already been achieved there.[18] The root problem underlying ongoing polio transmission is poverty, not lack of vaccination. Yet the Polio Eradication Initiative concentrates solely on immunization. In doing so, it draws attention away from political sources of inequality to focus on technical interventions (Ferguson 2006).

The Polio Eradication Initiative does not challenge global systems of inequality, and it is so narrowly focused on vaccination that it does not attempt to address other issues contributing to poliovirus circulation, such as poor sanitation. Yet I am not willing to condemn it for this reason. I have not yet seen a plan for the elimination of global inequality that is likely to be implemented. Improving sanitation across Pakistan is a slightly more achievable goal, and one that would have wide-reaching positive effects, but given the nation's high rates of population growth and urbanization, it is an extraordinarily tall order, and progress on this front has been incremental. If the Polio Eradication Initiative focuses on vaccination, the path of least resistance, it cannot be entirely faulted. Its planners know well the art of the possible.

Some scholars have argued that the efforts expended on polio eradication would have better been spent improving primary health care (Renne 2006). But the choice between eradicating polio and strengthening basic health services is not an either/or proposition. Polio eradication is a cause able to mobilize vast resources, such as the money provided by Rotary, that would likely not have been available for primary health care. Its narrow scope and technical focus are limitations, but not a priori reasons to condemn it.

I agree with the Polio Eradication Initiative officials who insist that polio eradication in Pakistan is "technically feasible." In Pakistan's belt of highest population density, the northern Punjab, with a string of megacities including Lahore, Gujranwala, Faisalabad, and Rawalpindi, polio was eliminated by 2004 (though it reappeared, imported from other areas of the country, in 2008). These extremely high-density cities, with high summer temperatures and poor sanitation, are ideal poliovirus habitat. Yet elimination has been achieved in these areas.

Key in stymieing the achievement of polio elimination, I believe, is what officials referred to as "management issues." Polio Eradication Initiative planners have done extensive analyses on what indicators correlate with districts that have ongoing poliovirus circulation and have come up with only a handful. Some are predictable—a lower number of doses of oral polio vaccine per child, more poorly covered areas during campaigns, higher population density—and not particularly revealing of underlying factors. The following more informative factors have been found to correlate significantly with ongoing polio transmission in a given district:

1)  Routine immunization coverage of less than 60 percent ($p = 0.001$) (Islamabad National Surveillance Cell data)
2)  Frequent transfers of the district health officer (aOR = 5.1, 95 percent CI = 1.03–25.5) (Lowther et al. 2002)
3)  Status as a "security-compromised area"; this indicator just missed statistical significance ($p = 0.066$) (Islamabad National Surveillance Cell data).

On the surface, these indicators are unrelated to one another, and all three do contribute to ongoing poliovirus transmission. Low routine immunization coverage means additional campaigns are needed to bring many children up to a baseline three doses of vaccine; frequent administrative transfers make for breaks in continuity; and insecurity makes planning and implementing campaigns difficult.

But none of these indicators alone should be sufficient to sustain poliovirus transmission. Districts with ongoing virus circulation are required to carry out subnational campaigns in addition to national campaigns—five extra in both 2007 and 2008—which should more than make up for subpar routine immunization rates. Even if district leadership changes, the procedures for carrying out polio vaccination campaigns remain the same, and the workers know the drill—there have been more than sixty campaigns thus far in Pakistan. Finally, as I discussed in the last chapter, fighting in all areas of Pakistan is sporadic, and while campaigns must sometimes be postponed in some areas they can almost always be carried out later.[19]

The significance of these indicators is that all of them are proxies for district health departments with poor accountability, voracious politics, and little commitment to the ideal of childhood immunization. These factors certainly contribute both to poor routine immunization coverage and to high rates of turnover in district administrations. They do not, of course, cause security problems in a district. However, these problems are compounded by insecurity. As I argued in the last chapter, lack of UN security clearance prevents WHO or UNICEF employees from traveling to insecure districts, leaving district health departments without the supervision and surveillance that these agencies use to pressure districts to implement quality vaccination campaigns. In insecure areas too other problems are likely to dwarf the threat of polio, and government employees may resist more tenaciously the suggestion that they risk their own safety to eradicate a disease that does not seem to be a major problem.

In short, a key reason—to my mind, the key reason—for ongoing poliovirus transmission in Pakistan is what planners in Islamabad called "management issues." Subsumed under this category were lack of actual (as opposed to spoken) commitment by health authorities from the village level to Islamabad, and what Polio Eradication officials called "inefficient utilization of human and financial resources" (and I called, in Chapter 4, corruption, patron-clientism, and refusal to work). In short, the difficulties the Polio Eradication Initiative faces in Pakistan are, I believe, primarily attributable to what I have described as a matrix of resistance on the part of government employees at a number of levels.

# Air Travel

The heat in Kaifabad is torrid in early June. Each evening the always weak electricity in my windowless house gives out entirely, and I can only pray there is enough water to stand in the shower with my clothes on in order to cool off enough to fall asleep. I board a crowded plane from Kaifabad to Abu Dhabi filled with migrant workers and give a huge sigh of relief: it is air-conditioned! When my second plane begins the descent into Geneva, circling around the sparkling lake ringed with snow-capped mountains, I feel I have entered an alternate universe.

Sarah is an American who works at the World Health Organization headquarters in Geneva.[1] She and her family live in an apartment in a village outside the city, where rolling green fields surround the small neighborhood shops. Her office—which has clearly not been renovated since the 1970s or earlier—is in the WHO complex, a cluster of buildings on a hill not far from the center of Geneva. It is served by a clean and reliable bus service, which she uses to get to work. Her daughter also takes public transportation to her private international school, a complex of beautifully restored old buildings on well-kept grounds whose fees of about $25,000 a year are paid by WHO. While her family enjoys living in Geneva, Sarah's job is hard on them; she is often gone more than two weeks out of every month.

Wherever she goes, Sarah stays in the best accommodations, which range from excellent in capital cities to questionable at best in the remote areas of Pakistan she visits to observe and monitor polio campaigns. I suspect the UN has a negotiated rate with the Islamabad Marriott, where she spends the most time when she is in Pakistan, but rates for the public there exceed two hundred dollars a night. She is able, there, to keep in touch with her office and family in Geneva via a broadband Internet connection, and exercise in the weight room or swim in the pool.

Sarah's job is demanding. When she is in Geneva, she regularly goes to the office on evenings and weekends, putting in close to seventy hours a week. When she is traveling, she may work more hours than that. She does it because she loves it, because it inspires her to be part of a historic goal like the eradication of polio, because she believes deeply that eradication is possible and that she has a responsibility to do everything she can to make it happen. She is thankful that WHO flies her business class so that she can get some sleep, but nonetheless she is often in a state of perpetual jet lag. She's so far into sleep debt, she says with a wan smile, that she's lost all hope of ever catching up.

# CHAPTER 6

# Geneva

I am an optimist.
—Bill Gates

## The Shift from International to Global Health

I BEGAN A MASTER's program in international health in 2003 but graduated in 2005 with a degree in global health.[2] The change in the moniker of my department reflected a larger trend: the term "global health" is replacing the previously dominant "international health" in the language of academics and bureaucrats working toward improving health in poor countries (Brown and Fee 2006). This change in appellation is intended to reflect the nature of disease in an increasingly globalized world, and to shift focus from individual nations to linkages across boundaries.

> While international health has sought to make systematic comparisons across national frontiers, global health views health and disease in a comprehensive, world-wide, integrated manner. This change in perspective on the world's health and health problems has emerged as a result of the establishment of newer and closer physical, economic, social, cultural, financial, and political linkages between nations, collectively referred to as globalization. One of the results of globalization is that morbidities and mortalities, once geographically unique, are no longer so confined. (Imperato 2001, 77)

The focus on global health carries with it an increased emphasis on the ideal of collaboration. This is framed as essential to the success of health initiatives in the new millennium: "Health problems today truly are global, and do not lend themselves to narrow parochial solutions. Cooperation, collaboration, and communication are more than a trendy shibboleth; they are ignored at the peril of genuine pandemic" (Banta 2001, 75).

Partnerships are the preferred mode of collaboration in this new global health. They provide a way of taking on projects too large for a single government or agency. The Global Alliance for Vaccines and Immunizations (GAVI); the Global Fund to Fight AIDS, Tuberculosis, and Malaria; the Stop TB Partnership; the Measles Initiative; and the Roll Back Malaria Partnership—all are extremely large partnerships that include some combination of multilateral and bilateral agencies, governments, and private-sector organizations. Many of these projects are modeled, more or less explicitly, on the Polio Eradication Initiative, the first global partnership of this type. In the current climate of collaboration, even partnerships need partners; for example, the Global Fund, itself a partnership, is listed as a partner of the Roll Back Malaria Partnership.

This proliferation of partnerships marks an important conceptual and cultural shift in the field of what is now global health. The conceptualization of the relationship between organizations such as the World Health Organization and the governments of poor countries like Pakistan as "partnership" and "collaboration" has important implications for the ability of international organizations to exert the power needed to carry out ambitious goals like eradication. The extent to which the culture of global health differs from the culture of international health thirty years ago, and the implications of this cultural shift, are clear when one compares the methods of the Polio Eradication Initiative to the single successful attempt at eradication, the Smallpox Eradication Program.

## The Smallpox Era

The last naturally occurring case of smallpox was that of a Somali cook in 1977.[3] The eradication of smallpox is widely and justifiably regarded as one of the great achievements of international health, cited by thinkers of widely divergent philosophies as an example of the best of international assistance (Easterley 2006, 242; Sachs 2005, 260). In the world of development, where progress is often all too elusive, smallpox eradication was an unqualified success.

Many of the challenges would-be smallpox eradicators faced were similar to those that have proven so formidable in the attempt to eradicate polio. The following description of the Pakistani government's efforts in smallpox eradication details problems different in specifics, but not in nature, from the obstacles to eradicating polio in that country:

By December 1968 major problems had become apparent. The government did not increase the budget [as it had promised] but, in fact, decreased it by 30%—to 1 million rupees. The plan envisaged the use of local body vaccinators as part of the complement of personnel but they were responsible to their own union councils (administrative units each responsible for a population of about 10,000) and the councils, in turn, to the Ministry of Basic Democracy. As the WHO adviser was to report: "A number of vaccinators have been appointed under political pressure and many of them are recommended by influential persons and are engaged in other duties or private jobs." . . . The Ministry of Basic Democracy was, with difficulty, persuaded to issue an order to the union councils directing local body vaccinators to work with the programme, an order which was subsequently ignored as often as it was respected. (Fenner et al. 1988, 691)

In short, World Health Organization representatives attempting to carry out smallpox eradication in Pakistan encountered government resistance of the type I described in Chapter 4: foot-dragging, false compliance, and patron-clientism.

Government officials in other countries also resisted WHO mandates. Lawrence Brilliant, who wrote a book on his experiences as a WHO employee in the Smallpox Eradication Program in India, noted that there were a few high-level government officials deeply committed to smallpox eradication, and that they and WHO officials in New Delhi formed a true team.[4] However, not all Indian government employees believed that smallpox eradication was an important goal. "However high a priority it was for the world community, as a whole smallpox eradication was not a priority for India so long as the number of cases appeared to be declining. The relative impact of smallpox [compared to other diseases] was negligible," Brilliant wrote. "Many policy makers felt that smallpox was more a priority for the United States or the USSR than for India" (Brilliant 1985, 30–33).

Nor were Indian officials convinced that the methods the World Health Organization advocated were the right way to go about smallpox eradication.[5] In at least one instance, the Indian minister of health publicly raised objections to World Health Organization methodology; despite these objections, immunization activities were carried out according to WHO's preferences. Thus it is not entirely surprising that government workers at all levels in India, aware of these disagreements, sometimes resisted carrying out their duties with the zeal that foreign WHO employees desired (Greenough 1995).

I have argued in this book that resistance on the part of government employees is the primary reason why polio is not yet eliminated in Pakistan. The question then arises: if there was resistance to smallpox eradication as well, how was smallpox eradicated? The primary reason is that, because of differences in the transmission of the viruses and the effectiveness of the vaccine, smallpox eradication was much easier than polio eradication. Most people gained immunity to smallpox after only a single dose of vaccine; in the case of polio in Pakistan, some children need as many as ten doses. Every case of smallpox was symptomatic, making it easy to trace transmission; there are hundreds of "silent" and untraceable polio infections for every person who develops paralysis. And, in contrast to the polio vaccine, the smallpox vaccine was effective even after people had already been exposed to smallpox, provided they had not yet developed symptoms.

There were also significant differences between the Smallpox Eradication Program and the Polio Eradication Initiative in the way WHO employees in each project dealt with resistance. The most striking difference lay in their approach to people who refused vaccination. In the Polio Eradication Initiative, people who refuse vaccination for their children are visited repeatedly by people attempting to persuade them to change their minds, but coercive tactics have, to my knowledge, never been used in Pakistan. At an orientation in Islamabad for some international workers sent by the CDC to work on polio eradication for three months, a man from Africa asked why police were not used to vaccinate refusals. His remark brought a few suppressed smiles.

"Constitutionally," a high-ranking Pakistani WHO official responded, "Pakistan is a democracy. . . . To me, the major issue is management; it's not really religious refusal."[6]

WHO officials in the Smallpox Eradication Program were less sanguine about refusals. Forcible vaccination of refusals was not official policy, but it was a fairly widespread practice by foreigners working for the program in South Asia (Greenough 1995). Lawrence Brilliant described one such encounter in India:

> In the middle of the gentle Indian night, an intruder burst through the bamboo door of the simple adobe hut. He was a government vaccinator, under orders to break resistance against smallpox vaccination. Lakshmi Singh awoke screaming and scrambled to hide herself. Her husband leaped out of bed, grabbed an ax, and chased the intruder into the courtyard.

Outside, a squad of doctors and policemen quickly overpowered Mohan Singh. The instant he was pinned to the ground, a second vaccinator jabbed smallpox vaccine into his arm.

Mohan Singh, a wiry 40-year-old leader of the Ho tribe, squirmed away from the needle, causing the vaccination site to bleed. The government team held him until they had injected enough vaccine; then they seized his wife. Pausing only to suck out some vaccine, Mohan Singh pulled a bamboo pole from the roof and attacked the strangers holding his wife.

While two policemen rebuffed him, the rest of the team overpowered the entire family and vaccinated each in turn. Lakshmi Singh bit deep into one doctor's hand, but to no avail. (Brilliant and Brilliant 1978)

There were, in fact, good reasons for smallpox eradicators to be more diligent than polio eradicators about covering refusals. I agree with the WHO official just quoted, who opined that refusals were a much less pressing issue in polio eradication than what he called "management" (and I have conceptualized as resistance). This is because of differences in the methods of the two programs. Smallpox eradication was achieved by creating a firewall of vaccinated people around each case of smallpox. A small pocket of refusals could derail the effectiveness of this strategy. Polio eradication, in contrast, depends on what epidemiologists call "herd immunity," or the immunity of the majority of the general population to polio.[7] In this approach, refusals are troubling but, so long as they remain a small percentage of the overall population, will not cause the strategy to fail.

Interestingly, one smallpox veteran I spoke with said that smallpox eradicators "became *less* coercive at the end," when they were ultimately successful. "We used force sometimes—and it didn't work," he said. The key to achieving high vaccination rates, in his opinion, was hiring health workers from infected villages, and not outsiders, to perform containment activities.

But foreign officials in the Smallpox Eradication Program in South Asia did not use coercive tactics only on people who refused vaccination. They also did their best to coerce unsupportive government officials into action. Often this took the form of exerting power they did not officially possess. For example, faced with the prospect of a city that was exporting large amounts of smallpox to other areas of India, Lawrence Brilliant placed the city under quarantine, ordering all buses and cars entering the city to be stopped and everyone inside vaccinated. Similarly, trains were kept away from the central station, and disembarking passengers were checked to make sure they were vaccinated (Brilliant and Brilliant 1978). What is most striking about this episode is not the quarantine but the fact that a foreigner took it upon himself to do what he felt needed to be done, regardless of the extent of his formal powers. One commentator wrote of Brilliant that "as a United Nations employee, he had no legal authority to close the city, but he did so by force of will, inspired by idealism and youthful daring" (Tucker 2001, 104).

Lawrence Brilliant was not alone in possessing this particular brand of chutzpah. In early 1975, the Smallpox Eradication Program in Bangladesh was in crisis. India and Pakistan had eliminated smallpox, but cases continued to occur in Bangladesh, nearly four thousand of them in April 1975 (Fenner et al. 1988). The situation was perilous because the secretary of health was considering abandoning the strategy of searching for cases and vaccinating around them, the surveillance-containment that had been so successful elsewhere, and returning to the less effective strategy of mass vaccination:

> [The secretary of health's] personal experience with smallpox control in the Ministry had been confined to the period since Bangladesh's independence, and for the last 4 years optimism had been expressed by the staff during and immediately after the monsoon each year, but epidemics and emergency programmes inevitably followed in the spring. For advice he turned most often to the WHO Representative in Bangladesh, a public health physician but one who understood neither smallpox epidemiology nor the eradication strategy any better than the Secretary of Health. With smallpox incidence rising and with increasing international interest as to whether Bangladesh could or would be able to stop transmission, tensions were great. The Secretary of Health and the WHO Representative repeatedly and vehemently demanded that the surveillance-containment programme should be stopped and the entire population vaccinated forthwith. (Fenner et al. 1988, 841–42)

Into the center of this dispute stepped D. A. Henderson, the head of the Smallpox Eradication Program in Geneva. A smallpox veteran who worked in Bangladesh told me: "When we were in real trouble, D. A. Henderson came from Geneva and threatened to quarantine the country, which he had no power to do, but it worked." (The WHO representative who advocated mass vaccination also left.) The strategy of surveillance-containment continued, and smallpox was eliminated from Bangladesh just six months later, in November 1975. Bangladesh's last smallpox case, and the world's last naturally occurring case of *Variola major,* the more virulent form of smallpox, was a girl of two and a half named Rahima Banu.

Such forceful actions are not the modus operandi in polio eradication. WHO officials in polio eradication know where the problems are and what would be required to rectify them, but they cannot take action to do so. Of course, officially the foreigners in smallpox eradication had no formal authority to do so either. But they did not let official rules get in the way of eradicating smallpox. If they felt coercion was necessary —whether of government employees or people who refused vaccination—they used it. This is a major difference in the cultures of the Polio Eradication Initiative and the Smallpox Eradication Program.

## Coercion and Success

I believe that the Smallpox Eradication Initiative's culture of using any means necessary, along with the fact that smallpox was epidemiologically easier to eradicate than polio, forms part of the explanation for its success. Eradication of a disease requires the simultaneous cooperation of people in all corners of every nation on earth. It is inevitable for would-be eradicators to encounter resistance in some areas, whether from recipient populations or the employees of delivery systems. Some of this resistance will be strong enough that standard techniques of social mobilization—radio and television advertisements, photo ops with high-ranking government officials—are insufficient to counter it. Coercive methods in certain times and places may be necessary. Coercion alone is certainly not a recipe for success in an eradication program; as the smallpox veteran quoted earlier observed, it is often not the best strategy. Malaria eradication's reliance on coercion rather than on productive relationships with potentially supportive recipient populations was a major weakness in its strategy (Packard 1997). But eradication is difficult; if it is to succeed, business as usual cannot be the modus operandi.

The longer an eradication program drags on, the more difficult success becomes. In polio eradication, planners often speak of "fatigue." In polio-endemic countries like Pakistan, workers have been told year after year that this year will be the last, that eradication is imminent and long hours and great attention to detail are needed *now*. These workers are tired and in many cases have lost faith. Workers in countries that have already eradicated polio are also prone to fatigue. Having eliminated polio through hard work, they must sustain extremely high vaccination coverage rates lest importations from polio-endemic countries undo their efforts. The longer they must do this, the harder it is to muster the enthusiasm—and the funding—for eradication.

In the case of smallpox, once activities were scaled up, the disease was eradicated quickly enough that fatigue did not present the problem it currently does in polio eradication. India, for example, went from around 190,000 cases of smallpox a year to zero in just twelve months (Brilliant 1985). This speedy eradication was possible primarily because of the epidemiology of smallpox and because the vaccine was so effective. However, coercive methods also played a part where resistance was present.

It is impossible to know what would have happened had smallpox eradication officials in places like Bangladesh not threatened government officials with punitive action. Perhaps smallpox would have been eradicated anyway. Or perhaps Bangladesh would have returned to mass vaccination and smallpox would have reinfected India, leading to a long, drawn-out campaign that ended in failure. The eradication of smallpox was far from a foregone conclusion; D. A. Henderson has said that it was "just barely" eradicated (Roberts 2006).

Eradication is such a difficult goal that it requires for its achievement the coming together of a large number of factors—and a good-sized dollop of luck. An excellent surveillance system, sufficient structural power to get all nations on earth to adopt the goal simultaneously, driven leadership—all are necessary to end forever the transmission of a disease that is in theory eradicable. More idiosyncratic factors may be important in certain times and places and not in others, including the ability to carry out eradication activities in the context of armed conflict, to adapt and create new strategies to deal with unique situations, to draw on the local knowledge of people living in places from Manila to Malawi, and to use coercion when necessary.

I am not arguing for the widespread use of coercive methods in eradication programs—even aside from the human rights concerns, they could certainly backfire. Paul Greenough has argued that the coercive methods used in smallpox eradication may have negatively affected other public health initiatives by turning public opinion against them (Greenough 1995). Nor can coercion play any productive role in control programs, which rely on long-term, sustainable strategies.[8] Nonetheless, for an eradication program, with its demand for compliance across large portions of the globe in a short time, some coercion may be necessary.[9]

Just because a particular goal is noble does not mean that everyone, everywhere, will enthusiastically support it. Some people, somewhere on earth, will always have political or religious reasons to object—or, as in the case of government workers in the Polio Eradication Initiative in Pakistan, little reason to give the program overwhelming support. Rhetoric of "partnership" or "collaboration," or the use of standard "social mobilization" programs, will not make these problems go away. If eradication is to be a public health goal—and, given the enthusiasm of Bill and Melinda Gates for the concept, it likely will be for some time—this objectionable truth must be dealt with. Honest discussion of the issues involved, and honest appraisal of what can be accomplished with the methods one is willing to use, would be a step in the right direction.

## Smallpox, Polio, and the Culture of Global Health

When they encountered resistance, Smallpox Eradication Program officials often used force. Polio Eradication Initiative officials tend to wait, proclaim loudly their faith and optimism, and hope things will change. Why was it that officials in the Smallpox Eradication Program felt free to use coercive methods while those in the Polio Eradication Initiative do not?

Some have opined that foreigners working on smallpox eradication were more likely to use coercive methods because they were isolated from supervision. It is certainly true that the introduction of cell phones has revolutionized communication in South Asia. When I arrived to do checking in an area where monitoring was supposed to be postponed, powerful officials were only a phone call away. Especially in remote areas where communication was previously slow, expensive, or nonexistent, the ability of lower-level employees to use cell phones provides an important check on foreigners' ability to use coercive methods.

But improved communications alone do not explain the relative absence of coercive methods in the Polio Eradication Initiative. If word reached officials in the Polio Eradication Initiative that a given foreign consultant was using coercive methods against refusals, no matter how belatedly they received that information, the person in question would likely be fired. (I have never heard of such behavior, as the use of coercive methods is simply out of the question.)

By contrast, there was a culture of rule breaking in the Smallpox Eradication Initiative that justified any means necessary to achieve the eradication of smallpox. Dr. M. I. D. Sharma, the acting commissioner of health for the Indian government and an active participant in smallpox eradication in India, prepared a "review of recipes for eradication of smallpox in India." These included "rules, regulations, and the routine breaking of rules and regulations" (Brilliant 1985, 146–147). The foreigners in the program were most likely to break rules because "there are risks in ignoring rules and breaking regulations, and the willingness to take those risks might have been greater in a temporary program that was not, for most of the participants, a lifetime career," Brilliant explains. "To some extent, experience from smallpox does corroborate an important aphorism: You can't make an omelet without cracking a few eggs" (Brilliant 1985, 155).

This culture of rule breaking differed from the overall culture of the World Health Organization at the time; Brilliant described the Smallpox Eradication Program as "what sociologist Max Weber has called a 'charismatic organization,' quite different from the formal organizational structure commonly associated with WHO." He also admitted that "an honest look at WHO in the postsmallpox years must acknowledge some degree of backlash against the zest of the eradicators" (Brilliant 1985, 71, 158).

To some degree, the culture of rule breaking in the Smallpox Eradication Program reflected the personality of its leadership. In his book on smallpox, Jonathan Tucker described the college years of D. A. Henderson, head of the Program:

> Tall and lanky (six feet, two inches), D. A. had a booming voice, an infectious grin, and an entrepreneurial spirit. He became editor of the college yearbook in his junior year, and he and his roommate founded a radio station that broadcast through the pipes of the campus heating system. They also devised creative strategies for bending the school rules. Although students were banned from having cars and everyone rode bicycles, there was no rule against motor scooters, which Henderson and his roommate used to zip around campus. Oberlin subsequently banned scooters but agreed to "grandfather in" the two young men on grounds of financial hardship. Exploiting another loophole, Henderson purchased a 1937 Oldsmobile as the "official car" of the college radio station. (Tucker 2001, 39–40)

But the credit, or blame, for the methods used in smallpox eradication cannot lie entirely with D. A. Henderson. Nor is it entirely plausible that the Smallpox Eradication Program was a total aberration, culturally different from most global public health projects before or since, especially when one considers that several of the highest-level officials in the Polio Eradication Initiative are smallpox veterans. Rather, I believe the primary reason for the difference in approach between the two programs is the shift in the larger culture of what used to be "international" and is now "global" health. The rhetoric of collaboration and partnership has real effects. As one global health practitioner put it to me, the "kind of containment strategies that worked" for smallpox "are not acceptable in today's public health world." The new paradigm, she opined, was "better from the point of view of respect," but worse when it came to meeting an ambitious goal like eradication.

## Power and Partnership

The increased focus on partnership, collaboration, and human rights in global health limits the exercise of power by agencies such as the World Health Organization, although no one in the Polio Eradication Initiative ever mentioned this to me as a burden or a limitation. The sort of methods used in the Smallpox Eradication Program simply never arose as a possibility in Pakistan. If they were suggested, as in the conversation with the visitor from Africa cited earlier, they were not taken particularly seriously. The ideals of collaboration and partnership, while fraught enough in practice, are sufficient to keep coercive methods from becoming a possibility.

But in addition to the arguably positive effect of limiting the coercion of officials or citizens of poor countries by employees of the World Health Organization, the rhetoric of partnership can work to obscure the power relations that do exist. As I argued in the last chapter, significant power was brought to bear on the Pakistani government to accept programs such as polio eradication and measles elimination. Yet because the relationship of the World Health Organization, UNICEF, and the Pakistani government is officially a partnership, its inherent difficulties and the resistance that employees of the Pakistani government present cannot be discussed openly at the policy level. WHO employees at all levels know what is happening; they are not deluded by the policy ideals. But in policy and planning, they have to hold tight to the fiction of Pakistani government partnership. The larger global health audience—donors, partners, ministers of health—demands that language. The World Health Organization provides it and in doing so ensures the continuation of the Polio Eradication Initiative.

This language has the dual effect of papering over the exercise of power by the World Health Organization and other multilateral and bilateral agencies, and of preventing open discussion in public forums about the nature of the problems polio eradication faces. Governments are presented as enthusiastic partners, which prevents a public admission that some governments are resisting the demands of the Polio Eradication Initiative. Because, in the official rhetoric, everyone is collaborating, serious public debate is out of the question regarding what would be necessary to achieve eradication, and the amount of power that organizations like the World Health Organization should be willing to exert.

The WHO officials working on polio eradication are of course very intelligent, and people based in Geneva know that the Pakistani government is a tenuous partner. Despite public proclamations that Pakistan was making progress and had government commitment, in private a WHO official in Geneva said what everyone inside the project knew: "hardly anything has improved; the underlying problem has not been addressed." The official added that the strategy of "hoping against hope that Musharraf is going to wake up and become a polio champion" had failed.

This is not to say that the hands of organizations like the WHO are tied. Even in the new era of global health, they retain significant leeway to exert structural power because the language of collaboration and partnership easily masks its use. They can pursue the goals of polio eradication and measles elimination in Pakistan, whose government is not enthusiastic about these programs. However, at the same time, international organizations are quite limited in their ability to use overt power, such as coercion, to take the steps necessary to complete the projects they have initiated. Thus the Polio Eradication Initiative remains marooned between success and failure, having achieved the miraculous through a combination of structural power, hard work, and actual collaboration, unable to exert quite enough influence to secure eradication.

## Donors, Skeptics, and the Big Muddy

In 2006, the smallpox veterans Isao Arita and Frank Fenner, along with Arita's colleague Miyuki Nakane, published an article in *Science* arguing that despite the "enormous benefit to mankind" represented by the Polio Eradication Initiative, "global eradication is unlikely to be achieved" (Arita, Nakane, and Fenner 2006, 852). They based their argument on the biological differences between polio and smallpox viruses and vaccines, and on the "greater degree of political independence" of many poor countries in the post–Cold War era (853). (Both the United States and the USSR supported smallpox eradication.) They also mentioned the long duration of the Polio Eradication Initiative as a factor inhibiting eradication. Accompanying their article was a more general news focus piece that quoted the skeptical views of several prominent figures in public health, among them D. A. Henderson, who was head of the Smallpox Eradication Program. "However diligent they are, however much the staff does its best, there are very serious obstacles that militate against eradicating polio," Henderson said (Roberts 2006, 832). In another interview, he said: "When we succeeded with smallpox, virtually all of my colleagues at the time felt that we had just barely made it. And there were so many positive things about smallpox eradication that made it so much easier than polio" (Thigpen 2004). Though Henderson was not listed as an author on the article by Arita, Nakane, and Fenner, he was rumored in polio eradication circles to have been behind it.

The news focus article also featured predictably optimistic statements from polio eradication leadership. David Heymann, the highest-ranking WHO official responsible for polio eradication, used the purported support of the governments of polio-endemic countries like Pakistan to argue for continuing the attempt at eradication: "As long as the partners and countries are willing to make the effort, it is not for Isao [Arita] or me to say that eradication is not feasible" (Roberts 2006, 835).

The WHO leadership's attempts at damage control notwithstanding, the sentiments expressed in the *Science* article, especially given the people quoted, posed a serious threat to the Polio Eradication Initiative. Both Isao Arita and D. A. Henderson had supported polio eradication at some point during the program (de Quadros 1997b; Roberts 2006). Their significant change of heart reinforced the doubts of many donors.

So grave were these doubts that by later that year, Pakistan's Polio Eradication Initiative was running out of money. Influenced by the *Science* article and their own misgivings, several major donors had begun scaling back their support for polio eradication. For example, JICA, the Japanese bilateral aid agency, which had provided between $8 million and $10 million for oral polio vaccine in Pakistan every year from 2000 to 2004, in 2005 reduced its vaccine funding to $6.5 million and in 2006 to $3.9 million. This reduction in funding, a representative of the agency told me, was due to the opinion of some Japanese officials that the program was a "failure." In late 2006, David Heymann visited Pakistan in a successful attempt to procure enough funding from donors to ensure the continuation of the program. During his visit, a WHO official with the *Science* article in his briefcase joked that he was carrying "dangerous literature."

By February of 2007, the monetary situation was desperate. Margaret Chan, the director-general of the World Health Organization, held an Urgent Stakeholders' Meeting in Geneva attended by government representatives of polio-endemic countries and representatives of major partners and donors, along with D. A. Henderson and Isao Arita. Framed as an opportunity to assess whether polio eradication was worth continuing, by most accounts the meeting was largely a festival of optimism; the PowerPoints presented were full of statements about "new approaches" (in the case of Pakistan, they referred to "new cross-border strategies," which were in reality only an incremental improvement over what had been going on for several years). "We can't give up now, was more of the feeling," someone who attended the meeting told me. I was also informed that Arita and Henderson remained largely silent.

The meeting succeeded in convincing high-level officials at key donor organizations to provide additional funding based on the likelihood of eradicating polio, thus granting the program a stay of execution. A representative of a bilateral donor agency in Islamabad told me that the result of the meeting was to "put a lot of pressure on us. . . . The meeting has done some—I don't know if it was good work." He added: "Otherwise we were not planning to provide" any funding in 2007.

But if bilateral donors were persuaded to give additional funding, they (aside from USAID, which was always supportive) also made it clear that they were skeptical about the effectiveness of that funding. The following exchange between a representative of a bilateral organization and a high-level representative of the World Health Organization took place at Pakistan's Technical Advisory Group in Islamabad a few months after the conference in Geneva. The donor representative was complaining that, although polio eradication appeared to be a well-run program, the expected date for eradication of polio from Pakistan had been pushed back three years in a row. Each year she was asked to come up with exceptional funding to help finish the job.

> Donor representative: I almost wish I hadn't believed you. . . . We also
>      have to be realistic—what if it doesn't happen? . . . Otherwise it's
>      very difficult to do it on a year-to-year ad hoc basis.
> WHO official: I can understand your disappointment. I hope you will
>      believe me—I think this year the target is more realistic—[mono-
>      valent vaccines] have not been widely tried yet. I do believe this
>      window of opportunity is more transparent. Have faith.[10]

At this meeting, a representative of the World Bank, another donor, stressed the need for a "three-year financing plan" with contingency plans for each year if polio was not eradicated. The government representatives at the meeting agreed to provide one. (Predictably, WHO employees in Islamabad were the ones who ultimately wrote it.)

A representative of one bilateral donor agency told me that they were concerned that polio eradication activities were, in addition to not eradicating polio, negatively influencing other immunization activities. Surveys showed various levels of routine immunization coverage across Pakistan. The survey used by Polio Eradication Initiative officials showed 77 percent coverage, but another survey, which the donor representative cited, showed only 50 percent coverage. "One reason may be—polio," he said, noting that time spent organizing and carrying out polio vaccination campaigns was time not spent on other health issues. "This is a difficult situation for us," he added. "We are still believing that there is a chance that this disease could be eradicated." This donor, like the Japanese, had scaled back its funding but not eliminated it entirely.

WHO officials in Geneva were acutely aware that they needed to make real progress—and soon—to keep donors on board. "Donors are tired," Bruce Aylward, the head of polio eradication at WHO, told the media. "And there's always a risk with goals and targets. We have four countries left. If three hit the goal, you are in good shape. If all four of them miss, people will want to take another hard look" (Donnelly 2007). A WHO employee I spoke to in Geneva was more direct: "If we don't finish *somewhere* by the end of the year, we're going to be screwed."

Ultimately, polio was not eradicated in any of the four endemic countries by 2007—or by 2008. Pakistan and Afghanistan were widely viewed as the closest to achieving eradication, but polio retained its tenacious hold in several areas of circulation. Yet the Polio Eradication Initiative was able to obtain enough funding to keep activities going. Even in the midst of the 2008–2009 global financial crisis several years later, polio eradication has found funding. Between August 2008 and March 2009, donors gave nearly $700 million—barely enough to keep the project running. Early in 2009, Bill Gates announced that he would donate $255 million if Rotary came up with another $100 million. He indicated that he was committed to polio eradication for the foreseeable future:

> Eradicating a disease is hard, slow, painstaking work. . . . If somebody says we'll eradicate polio tomorrow, they're wrong about the immediate future. But if somebody says we won't eradicate polio ever, they're wrong about the long term. We do not know when, but we do know that we will eradicate polio. . . . Either we eradicate polio, or we return to the days of tens of thousands of cases per year. That is no alternative at all. We don't let children die because it is fatiguing to save them. (Gates 2009)

Rotary clubs responded; the one I attend in rural Vermont raised nearly two thousand dollars for the cause by passing around a special donation jar at each meeting. There is no a priori reason to believe that the next few years will be better for polio eradication than the past few years, yet the Polio Eradication Initiative was able to secure the money it needed to continue its elusive quest.

One of the reasons polio eradication attracts donors is that the program is extraordinarily well run and tightly supervised. Donors can feel confident that the Polio Eradication Initiative will do what it says it will do—on schedule, and with careful monitoring. A representative of one bilateral donor told me: "We don't have to invent something to monitor it. It's easy." Another said: "It's meeting all the agreed outputs." Donors can give to polio eradication and know exactly where their money is going.

In choosing whether to continue supporting the project, these donors are engaging in a type of decision common enough, and fraught enough, to have a literature devoted to it. Polio eradication's end-stages are a classic case of what scholars of management call "escalation of commitment to a failing course of action."[11] Research and theory on this topic flourished in the aftermath of the Vietnam War. Studies—most of them conducted using undergraduates at U.S. universities—showed that people were more likely to pour larger investments into failing projects than into successful ones (Staw 1976). Scholars who wanted to know what drives people to invest additional resources in an endeavor that has thus far not yielded the expected benefits identified a number of factors that apply to polio eradication. People are especially likely to "throw good money after bad" when:

- Projects are perceived as being close to completion (Boehne and Paese 2000; Garland and Conlon 1998).
- There are large amounts of "sunk costs" already committed to the project. When (as in polio eradication) success of the project would allow someone to recoup these sunk costs and break even, the temptation to make additional investments is very strong. Several studies of gambling have shown that people who are losing badly become very reckless, looking for a potential payoff in an attempt to break even (Post et al. 2007; Thaler and Johnson 1990).
- Failures can be explained by external factors or flukes (Staw 1981). Though a cogent argument could be made for polio eradication's difficulties not being flukes at all, high-level leadership insisted that they were, as with the official in Geneva who told me that they had been "unlucky."
- The person making the decision about whether to allocate additional resources is the same person who initially decided to embark on the failing course of action (Brockner 1992; Staw 1981). This

effect is especially strong when the person in question is insecure in their job or defending an unpopular position (Fox and Staw 1979). People who need to justify the initial decision to pursue a goal are more likely to make extreme gambles in the hope that it succeeds.

The end-stages of an eradication program seem tailor-made to exacerbate this "knee-deep in the big muddy" phenomenon. Because these end-stages are the most difficult, failure is likely to come at the point when, as in polio eradication, the project is "a 99.9% success," as Musharraf put it, and when vast amounts of energy and money have already been invested.

In the case of polio eradication, the World Health Organization has its professional reputation riding on success. The WHO no longer occupies the global leadership role on global health issues it once enjoyed. In the late 1990s, it was, according to some observers, an "organization in crisis" (Brown and Fee 2006, 62), able to survive only by entering partnerships with the new major global health players such as the World Bank and the Gates Foundation. While polio eradication is not exclusively a WHO program, its global leadership works out of Geneva and failure of the project would be a heavy blow to the WHO.

## Optimism Revisited

The optimistic statements prepared by the World Health Organization in which governments are said to be committed, new vaccines are touted as breakthroughs, and eradication is ever imminent are in part calculated attempts to keep donors on board. The more skeptical donors become, the more resolutely optimistic employees of the World Health Organization feel they have to be to ensure that they have the money to keep on going. Sometimes, a few WHO employees told me, they deliberately take a "glass half full" approach.

That said, the optimism in the World Health Organization is not simply calculated. There is a deep culture of optimism in the Polio Eradication Initiative there, and people I spoke to at the highest levels of leadership genuinely believed, it seemed to me, that eradication of polio was just around the corner. Whether one views this as commitment to a vision or, in the words of a CDC employee, as "self delusion," this culture of optimism has concrete implications for the course of polio eradication. It was probably necessary to get polio eradication off the ground and is not

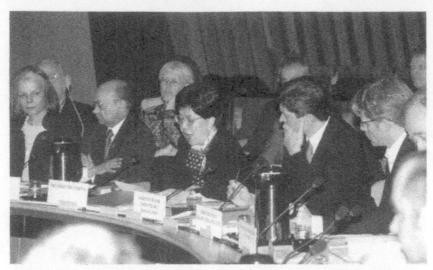

The highest-level leaders of the Polio Eradication Initiative meet at the WHO Headquarters in Geneva in 2007. In the front row, from left: Julie Gerberding, Director of CDC; Kul Gautam, Deputy Executive Director of UNICEF; Margaret Chan, Director-General of the World Health Organization; David Heymann, WHO Representative of the Director-General for Polio Eradication; and Bruce Aylward, Director of the Polio Eradication Programme at WHO. Photo: WHO/Chris Black.

irrelevant in polio eradication's ability to keep donors hooked. But it has less positive effects as well.

Most crucially, the culture of optimism prevents hard-nosed, objective analysis of what would be necessary to achieve polio eradication. It fosters the appealing but naïve assumption that because a goal is worthy, it will find support in all corners of the globe. It allows planners to avoid dealing with the most intractable problems of resistance and insecurity by explaining away failures as bad luck. In short, by preventing open discussion and debate about the very real difficulties the project faces, the culture of optimism contributes to polio eradication's current quagmire.

The current climate of global health, with its emphases on partnership and collaboration, provides particularly fertile ground for unbridled optimism to grow. Part of the culture of optimism is allowing global health's language to stand as if it represented reality. By recasting reluctant governments as "partners" and disgruntled workers as "volunteers," the lexicon of global health assists in obscuring from public view the real problems of resistance.

Eradication is a Utopian project, and a strong dose of optimism is nec-

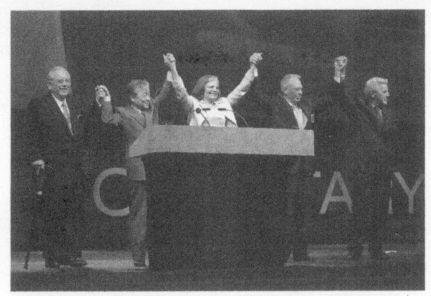

The culture of optimism: The leaders of the major partners in the Polio Eradication Initiative at the 2005 Rotary convention. Polio was to have been eradicated by 2005, so from one perspective the program had failed. From left to right: Glenn Estes Sr., Rotary president; Lee Jong-Wook, WHO Director-general; Julie Gerberding, CDC Director; Carlo Ravizza, Rotary Foundation chairman; Louis-Georges Arsenault, UNICEF. Photo: © 2009 Monika Lozinska-Lee/Rotary Images.

essary to attempt it. Historically, the culture of optimism has been strong in all of the World Health Organization's major eradication programs. Lawrence Brilliant wrote of a "climate of optimism" among the WHO employees of the Smallpox Eradication Program (Brilliant 1985, 30). The historian Randall Packard points out that malaria eradication was characterized by a postwar "optimism about our ability to transform the world" (Packard 1997, 289).

And not only would-be disease eradicators are optimistic. Development projects generally are driven by faith in the idea that transcending poverty and sickness is possible and, given enough money, immanent.[12] Celebrity economist Jeffrey Sachs, one of the architects of the Millennium Development Goals, "reject[s] the plaintive cries of the doomsayers who say that ending poverty is impossible" (Sachs 2005, 328). Sachs's message is that poverty can be ended, worldwide, given enough development aid. Sachs's voice—one that refuses to let rich countries make excuses about our abysmal failure to assist the poor—is a useful one. His arguments are appealing to potential donors. But poverty will not, as he claims it can, be eradicated by 2025.

Optimism in development is a double-edged sword, a necessary evil. It is a very useful tool in procuring money. It permits attacks on problems that would otherwise seem impossible. The danger comes when that optimism undercuts those very projects by preventing stern analysis of the problems they face, and what would be necessary to overcome these problems. When optimism leads, as in the case of Sachs, to a dismissal of the impact of the legacy of colonialism and of ongoing patterns of exploitation, it is safe to predict that problems wait in the wings. When, as in the case of polio eradication, optimism prevents planners from acknowledging the power relationships they bump up against daily, a quagmire results.

The way forward is not to abandon hope about the ends, but to become more realistic about the means. There are no simple solutions to the complexities of implementation in global health projects. The elites who control the governments of many poor countries like Pakistan have little reason to make the health of the poor their first priority, especially given the pressing demands from other quarters. One alternate strategy—bypassing the government entirely and working through NGOs—has its own set of problems, beginning with how it may weaken health systems (Pfeiffer 2004). These dilemmas have no easy answers and no perfect solutions.

The unfortunate current modus operandi in global health, driven by the synergistic demands of the culture of optimism and the need to please donors, is to frame the fraught power relationships between funders, planners, and implementers in terms of partnership and collaboration. This allows imperfect projects to continue but otherwise serves no one well: not the donors who want their money to make an impact, the people who devote their lives to working toward improvement in global health, or, most importantly, the poor and sick.

## The End of the Line

I walk to Zainab's house from my house in Kaifabad
through streets not wide enough for a car, redolent with
raw sewage from the open gutters that run down both
sides of the road. None of the houses in her neighborhood
has a yard. They all share three walls with other homes,
the fourth wall flush with the narrow alleyway. Most of
the houses are two stories, with one extended family on
each floor.

Zainab lives on the ground floor of a small house
with her husband's parents, his three brothers, and their
families. I have never counted how many children live in
this space, but their enthusiasm always overwhelms me as
they pull me through their gate into their tiny, rundown
entryway and attempt to force their beleaguered parrot
to perform a new word for me. Some of the children are
usually preparing potatoes to be made into french fries at
Zainab's brother-in-law's tiny and struggling storefront
shop.

Zainab's room, which she shares with her husband
and six children, is barely large enough for the heavy
and ornately carved bed and dresser that were her
dowry. (Some of the older children sleep in the extended
family's shared living room.) Her husband is a driver in a
government office and makes Rs. 10,000 (about $160) a
month—not enough for Zainab to afford a separate home
for her family. As always, Zainab seats me on the bed,
plumps the pillows around me, and goes to make me tea.
In this female space, Zainab's younger sisters-in-law and
I allow our cotton *dupaṭṭās*, or headscarves, to fall off our
heads while we talk. They are both fairly recently married,

and still wearing the fancy clothing that was in their bridal trousseaus.

Over milk tea, biscuits, samosas, and french fries (Zainab is always a generous hostess), I turn on my audio recorder and interview Zainab about the immunization of her children. Of the six, two are under five. Zainab has made sure that both of them got their full course of routine immunizations. Her young children also received polio drops in the last door-to-door campaign. Zainab, a talkative woman, readily elaborates on anything she can think of having to do with polio immunization:

> The woman who comes to our house to give polio drops, she's become my friend. Even if I'm not here, she'll make sure she gives my children the polio drops before she leaves. Whenever she comes, especially in the winter, she'll have a cup of tea here. She's a good woman [*ek acchi mohazab si 'aurat hai*]. There's a young girl who comes with her.

And there you have it: the most detailed, in-depth conversation about the polio campaigns I had with any of the seventy-eight mothers I interviewed. Zainab believes that vaccination is a good thing; she has gotten to know the woman who came door-to-door delivering polio vaccine; really, what more is there to say?

# CHAPTER 7

# Conclusion

A world free of measles by 2015 is not a dream.
—Ciro de Quadros

We have a real chance to build the partnerships, generate
the political will, and develop the scientific breakthroughs
we need to end this disease. We will not stop working until
malaria is eradicated.
—Bill Gates

Any goal short of eradicating malaria is accepting malaria.
It's making peace with malaria. It's rich countries saying,
we don't need to eradicate malaria around the world as
long as we've eliminated it in our own countries. That is
just unacceptable.
—Melinda Gates

The field of global public health is currently in an era of unprecedented
funding and ambitious goal making.[1] The global financial crisis of 2008–
2009 is likely to have some effect on aid (McNeil 2009), but it takes place
in the context of historically high levels of funding for global health initiatives: $21.8 billion in 2007, compared to $5.6 billion in 1990 (Ravishankar et al. 2009). It is not surprising that, in this climate, the ideal of
eradication would find supporters. The World Health Organization and
other major global health funders and organizations are poised to attempt
massive eradication efforts targeting measles and—shockingly, to many
observers including myself—malaria.

Like the Polio Eradication Initiative on which it is modeled, the
Measles Initiative started with a disease elimination campaign in the
Americas. In 1994, riding the crest of the successful elimination of polio in
the Americas, and inspired by the successful elimination of measles from
several countries in the Caribbean, the Pan American Sanitary Conference

moved to eliminate measles from the Americas by 2000 (Pan American Health Organization 1994). Their strategy of mass measles campaigns was modeled in important ways on polio campaigns and made use of the infrastructure created by polio elimination efforts (Acharya et al. 2002; Hersh et al. 2000). These efforts were quite successful, reducing the number of cases from hundreds of thousands per year to just a handful (de Quadros et al. 2004).[2] In 2001, the Measles Initiative began efforts to replicate this success globally (Hoekstra et al. 2006). It made great progress, reducing yearly measles deaths by a reported 74 percent worldwide by 2007 (Measles Initiative 2009).

The Measles Initiative has not declared itself an eradication program and probably will not do so if polio eradication is not achieved. However, people involved in the project—many of whom were instrumental in launching the Polio Eradication Initiative—have indicated that if polio is eradicated, they want measles to be next. A number of recent articles have argued that measles eradication is "technically feasible" (de Quadros et al. 2008; Fenner 1999; Meissner, Strebel, and Orenstein 2004; Orenstein et al. 2000). The Measles Initiative's leaders seem to regard polio eradication as a test case. "Launching a global initiative on measles eradication will require demonstrating that polio has been eradicated," writes Ciro de Quadros, an influential leader in both the polio and measles elimination efforts in the Americas (de Quadros 2004, 137). The eradication of polio would provide excellent impetus to push the Measles Initiative, which has made substantial headway in reducing measles mortality worldwide, into high gear (Orenstein et al. 2000).

In contrast, the malaria eradiation project, proposed by Bill and Melinda Gates in 2007, is a new effort, at this point a concept rather than a reality. But would-be eradicators of malaria are hoping that the eradication of polio will give their project a boost. Bill Gates said: "We're very committed to polio because we think success there will breed positive excitement. A failure there would definitely be a setback for malaria and all diseases. Just the whole idea of success would seem so remote that that would hurt a lot." However, he immediately added: "Our commitment [to malaria eradication] won't wane no matter what happens in this area. It's a lifetime commitment on our part. And, I do think people will join in" (Gates and Gates 2007). Malaria eradication, then, will probably remain a goal no matter what happens in the course of polio eradication.

The lessons of polio eradication could prove critical for these two very big, very ambitious, very difficult projects. I have argued in this book that the need to frame projects in a way that impresses donors and faith in the power of technological solutions to health problems contribute to a culture of optimism in the World Health Organization. The problems experienced by the Polio Eradication Initiative grow out of this culture of optimism, which fosters the unrealistic expectation that polio eradication will be a priority in every district in every nation of the world simultaneously. The ideals of participation and collaboration that drive current global health policy are part of this culture and hide the exercise of power by UN agencies behind a rhetoric of partnership. Officials at places like the World Health Organization in Geneva—themselves constrained by the language and ideals of partnership—have no direct control over the implementation of immunization activities and are unable to make polio the only priority in a nation beset with more politically pressing problems. Meanwhile, it falls to highly political district health bureaucracies and workers to implement the kind of near-perfect polio vaccination campaigns required for achieving eradication. These government workers, besieged by local political maneuvering and frustrated by their poor pay, resist the mandates of the Polio Eradication Initiative with strategies such as foot-dragging, false compliance, and a reliance on networks of patron-clientism.

Like the Polio Eradication Initiative, the projects aiming to eradicate measles and malaria are characterized by optimism and a belief in the possibilities of partnership. It is likely, then, that they will face the same problems of resistance that have presented such a challenge to the eradication of polio and will be similarly ill equipped to handle them. In this chapter, I consider the challenges measles and malaria eradication efforts face and present concrete suggestions for making planning for these projects better.

## Optimism and the Challenge of Eradication

Perhaps the most important cautionary tale that the Polio Eradication Initiative offers is that eradication of a disease in the current global political system is extremely difficult. Yes, the eradication of smallpox was successful, but the programs aiming to eradicate polio, measles, and malaria face challenges of a different order. First, the biological and epidemiological characteristics of the smallpox virus and the nature of the vaccine made the eradication of smallpox easier than that of any of the currently targeted diseases. But perhaps even more importantly, smallpox eradication took place in a different era, that of late-stage colonialism and the Cold War. Smallpox eradication was originally championed by the USSR and gained traction when the United States agreed to throw its weight behind the project (Fenner et al. 1988). The combined structural power of the United States and the USSR at that moment in time, within the sudden power vacuum of a recently decolonized world, would probably dwarf the power of any organization or partnership in the current era of globalization. On what has become such a fragmented and complex world stage, eradication may be impossible.

Part of the culture of optimism is faith that governments will be eager collaborators in eradication programs. The projects targeting measles and malaria rely heavily on the ideals of partnership and collaboration that I argue have prevented polio eradication planners from addressing their problems head-on. While the project of malaria eradication is too new to have an explicit structure, Bill and Melinda Gates, in announcing their commitment to eradication, have called for partnership from entities as diverse as governments, UN agencies, NGOs, and corporations. Bill Gates opined that where governments are not sufficiently committed to malaria eradication, the solution was yet more partnership, the creation of coalitions of governments. "Helping strengthen some of these African based regional groups and continent wide groups may be an important part of the fight against malaria" (Gates and Gates 2007).

The Measles Initiative is a partnership explicitly modeled on the Polio Eradication Initiative and includes many of the same players—WHO, UNICEF, and the CDC. (The major difference is the private-sector partner: in the Measles Initiative, it is the Red Cross, not Rotary.) The Measles Initiative in Pakistan is being carried out by precisely the same people as the Polio Eradication Initiative, as noted earlier, and the Measles Initiative already faces the problems of resistance that have made the eradication of polio so difficult there.

Epidemiologically, polio is a far more difficult disease to eradicate than smallpox, but measles would be harder still (Elliman and Bedford 2007). The measles vaccine is effective, but achieving high levels of immunity in poor countries requires several injections, and measles is highly infectious (de Quadros 2004; Griffin and Moss 2006; Meissner, Strebel, and Orenstein 2004; Orenstein et al. 2000). While the elimination of polio from the Americas has proved fairly durable, the elimination of measles has been tough to maintain—the importation of cases from other areas of the world is ongoing.[3] Even in Europe, the elimination of measles has proved elusive, largely because of low vaccination coverage in several countries, including Switzerland and Germany (Muscat et al. 2009). For these reasons, not everyone agrees that measles eradication is a reasonable goal: one measles expert was recently quoted as saying that measles eradication was "just not feasible" (Childs 2007).

While the probability of measles eradication remains questionable, the eradication of malaria is widely agreed to be impossible. Even malaria eradication's most fervent supporters admit that the tools to eradicate malaria are not currently available—although they have faith that these will be developed through new research and thus are pushing ahead. "We'll use today's tools today," one enthusiast said, "and tomorrow's tools tomorrow" (McNeil 2008). The rationale of the Gates Foundation is that setting the currently impossible goal of eradication will spur scientific breakthroughs that will make it attainable (Okie 2008). Skeptics point out that not only is malaria not eradicable with the current means, but that we may actually lose some tools to insecticide and drug resistance (Kelly-Hope, Ranson, and Hemingway 2008; Mendis et al. 2009).[4]

The rebirth of optimism about malaria eradication is striking, given that the midcentury malaria eradication program was one of the more spectacular failures in the history of global public health. The negative aftereffects of the failure lingered for years. In the decades after the World Health Organization gave up on malaria eradication and switched its goal to control, there was a resurgence of the disease.[5] Funding for malaria decreased, and malaria research slowed (Brown 1997). D. A. Henderson reported that one planner felt "the program had done a far better job in eradicating malariologists than malaria" (Henderson 1999, S55).

The revitalization of the malaria eradication concept signals a worrisome resistance to learning from the past. In her speech advocating malaria eradication as a global health goal, Melinda Gates mentioned the earlier eradication attempt but explained away its serious problems: "The world wasn't ready for a long fight" (Gates and Gates 2007).

Despite the daunting challenges facing malaria eradication, many of the major players in global health have embraced it. Immediately after Bill and Melinda Gates announced eradication as a goal, Margaret Chan, director-general of the World Health Organization—invoking polio eradication as a model—promised the support of the WHO (reportedly without first discussing the issue with some of the people who would be involved) (Roberts and Enserink 2007). "I . . . pledge WHO's commitment to move forward with all of you," Chan announced at the Bill and Melinda Gates Foundation Malaria Forum. "And, I dare you to come along with us" (Chan 2007c).[6] Her jaunty enthusiasm was mirrored in other responses to the Gates announcement. The editors of the influential journal *Lancet*, for example, wrote that "only by setting our collective sights higher will we make the progress we know we can make against malaria" (*Lancet* 2007, 1459). In fact, the influence of the Gates Foundation is so great that many people who believe, with good reason, that malaria eradication is impossible reportedly feel reluctant to voice that opinion publicly (McNeil 2008). This phenomenon has even acquired a name—the "Gates

Effect" (Roberts and Enserink 2007)—and represents a form of structural power all its own. The optimism necessary to launch an eradication program against a disease not eradicable with existing methods is, from my perspective, stunning.

It is my position that the programs attempting to eradicate measles and malaria are ill advised. If polio *is* eradicated, planners should thank their lucky stars, give health staff across the world a well-deserved week-long paid vacation in lieu of yet another vaccination campaign, and hang the eradication concept up on the wall until the development of a different world system or a bona fide magic bullet. The chances of either the measles or malaria eradication program succeeding are slim, and the impacts of their failure would be significant.

I am unable to advocate abandoning polio eradication, because of the real dangers of the failure of such a large eradication program, along with heartache for the enormous amount of work that millions of people have put into the project. Proponents of ending the Polio Eradication Initiative have called for a return to "effective control," defined as less than five hundred cases per year globally (Arita, Nakane, and Fenner 2006, 853). But this is an unrealistic strategy for polio in India and Pakistan, where the current program of near-monthly door-to-door campaigns barely keeps polio under "control." In the absence of a global eradication effort, neither the funding nor the motivation for these recurring campaigns would be forthcoming. The current high levels of population immunity would evaporate.[7] Polio cases in South Asia would probably leap quickly to thousands each year, and importations to other areas of the globe would likely be inevitable. As in the case of the midcentury malaria eradication program, the failure of polio eradication would likely have serious repercussions.

## The Problem of Resistance

Many working in polio eradication in Islamabad blamed the failures of the project on "management issues," usually the inability or unwillingness of district health officials to ensure that their employees carried out polio eradication activities with the level of attention to detail necessary. They were referring to situations like one I have described, where ensuring a high-quality immunization campaign did not appear to be the district health leadership's only or primary goal (see Chapter 3).

The importance of this issue of management in global health in general and eradication in particular is often noted (Foege et al. 2005). Halfdan

Mahler, then WHO's director-general, called smallpox eradication "a triumph of management, not of medicine" (Bate 2007, 102). After achieving smallpox eradication, D. A. Henderson, head of the Smallpox Eradication Program, called for the global eradication of "bad management" (J. Hopkins 1989, 134). Smallpox veteran Bill Foege wrote that "the lack of management skills appears to be the single most important barrier to improving health throughout the world" (Foege 2005, xvi).

At a basic level, to be a good manager one must have the ability to organize, lead, and motivate one's staff. But lack of ability at the district level was not what made polio eradication so difficult, although there were probably cases in which leaders were simply ineffective or disorganized. (In any case, the World Health Organization had international consultants in nearly every district to conduct activities like planning.)

The problem was resistance from the district health leadership and their employees, including doctors, vaccinators, lady health workers, and volunteers. Where district leaders were unable to control their staff, this was often because they were facing widespread resistance from employees angry about pay or the demands placed on them. And district health leaders themselves often resisted the imposition of international mandates.

Part of my strategic advice for avoiding polio eradication's morass is to recognize, name, and plan around resistance. As I have argued, resistance is a matrix of diffuse and disorganized behaviors—including foot-dragging, false compliance, and reliance on patron-client networks rather than on formal structures of authority—which taken together can derail the plans of superiors. My insistence on calling these behaviors "resistance" may seem to be a matter of semantics, but a shift in labeling from "bad management" (or, as I discuss later, "lack of political will") to "resistance" may yield important changes in the way these problems are dealt with. Thinking about them as "resistance" forces an admission that advocacy, social mobilization, and other methods of persuasion will do little to change the patterns of behavior that stymie eradication, and that perhaps what is needed is an entirely different approach.

## The Way Forward

People outside the Polio Eradication Initiative often ask me whether the answer to polio eradication's problems is increased community participation. Tapping into grassroots support for polio eradication, this reasoning goes, could overcome the resistance by government employees. At some level, this assumption is correct. For instance, smallpox eradication veterans have told me that working with local communities was key to eradicating the disease in India.

The problem is that polio is not a ranking public health problem in Pakistan. In a country where one in ten children dies before age five, polio now paralyzes fewer than a hundred children each year. Also, polio's status in Pakistan as an endemic, not an epidemic, disease means that it does not evoke the fear that it did in the midcentury United States. In the case of smallpox eradication, community participation was sought when active cases of smallpox were in the vicinity—when anyone around could understand the danger. Polio eradication, which relies on mass vaccination of the entire population, cannot rely on the fear of parents around a single polio case to galvanize nationwide vaccination.

Polio eradication planners do their best. When I was in Pakistan, they launched a major social mobilization campaign of polio true stories hosted by a popular television personality. These spots told the life stories of people handicapped by polio, usually ending with a key message delivered by the polio survivor. These spots were well received by the mothers I knew. But in a world with myriad other health threats—not to mention the question of how to make meager incomes stretch to cover food, clothing, and school fees—polio immunization was, while widely viewed as a good thing, simply not a priority for most women. They accurately assessed the threats to their children, and polio did not make the top of the list. Nor should it have. It was a priority disease only for those who were trying to eradicate it. Community willingness was not a problem. But community participation was not, and would never be, forthcoming.

These realities are often cited in arguments against vertical programs like eradication, which may be divorced from the needs of their putative beneficiaries, and in favor of the primary health care model, which aims to involve the recipients of health care initiatives in setting agendas and implementing projects.[8] The debate between proponents of vertical and community-based programs is one of long standing. I confess I began my fieldwork with a prejudice against vertical programs, but as I saw in greater detail how the Polio Eradication Initiative worked, I became to some degree a convert. The narrow focus and clear goals of polio eradication allowed a level of accountability which, while not perfect, was far greater than that in the more diffuse, putatively community-based projects I had observed in the country. Because the project had clear benchmarks and clear, measurable standards, people could be held responsible for the quality of their work. This accountability was not total, as we have seen, and not sufficient to rapidly secure the elimination of polio from the country. Still, the quality of work in polio eradication was better than that in any other government health initiative I have observed in Pakistan. Of course, reliable, functioning primary health care is the ultimate goal. But vertical programs have the significant benefit of being able to implement key interventions quickly even in areas where village-level health provision is in shambles.

Thus, while I would argue against the adoption of another eradication program, the judicious use of vertical programs—in combination with programs based in the primary health care model—can ensure the delivery of key interventions. The Global Alliance for Vaccines and Immunizations (GAVI), which funds routine immunization in Pakistan, is one example of such a program. It aims to ensure that 90 percent of Pakistan's children receive the full course of routine immunizations. This project, like an eradication program, has clear goals and easily measurable indicators. Unlike polio eradication—viewed by many at the district level as something of a wild goose chase—routine immunization coverage is widely viewed as an important goal by health staff. The GAVI system includes most of the same players as polio eradication and is probably subject to some resistance as well. Its ambitious goal of 90 percent routine immunization coverage is unlikely to be attained. But since it is not an eradication program, even if it does not meet its stated goals, it can still claim a measure of success.

Eradication programs are risky ventures in a world in desperate need of proven solutions. If eradication programs are to be attempted (and I think it would probably be better if they were not), it is important that the potential barriers to eradication—and what would be necessary to overcome them—are clearly conceptualized and planned for. I offer two key suggestions for planners of eradication programs: a precommitment analysis of political feasibility and a program for designing adaptive flexibility into the end-stages of an eradication program.

## Political Feasibility

Assessments of technical and operational feasibility are often used to predict whether a given disease is eradicable. Technical feasibility refers to the biologic characteristics of the disease and the effectiveness of the tools we have to fight it, but not to issues like logistics, the existence of delivery systems, or the disruption caused by events like war. The eradication of polio and measles are generally considered technically feasible (Losos 1999). The eradication of malaria is not.

Operational feasibility refers to the capacity of systems to deliver the necessary interventions to the necessary places in order to achieve eradication. The Polio Eradication Initiative is a testament to the ability of copious funding and international pressure to make a project operationally feasible. Polio eradication requires a cold chain of refrigeration to deliver fresh vaccine door-to-door in the remotest corners of the earth. It requires trained doctors acting as surveillance personnel in every part of the globe, with the transportation and equipment to reach, in short order, any family, anywhere, whose child becomes paralyzed. It requires a global network of laboratories with the staff and equipment to take stool samples from those paralyzed children (delivered rapidly through yet another cold chain) and quickly determine whether the children were infected with poliovirus and, if so, of what type. On paper, this would all have seemed impossible in a place like Pakistan, and yet it has all been achieved and is functioning extraordinarily well. In a year working on polio eradication in Pakistan, for example, I never saw a single vial of vaccine whose heat-sensitive label indicated a break in the cold chain. The logistical structure of the Polio Eradication Initiative in Pakistan was nothing less than a miracle of planning and funding. The problems polio eradication faces are not operational in the sense that, in the words of one WHO official, the WHO and its international partners had been able to put all the "necessary enabling factors" in place.

Polio eradication planners have claimed that the term "operational feasibility" encompasses not just logistics but "societal and political considerations" (Aylward, Hull, et al. 2000, 285). The argument in this book is that it is *precisely* societal and political considerations that are preventing polio eradication from being successful. Yet polio eradication leadership insists that the "operational feasibility of achieving it has been demonstrated under every circumstance imaginable" (ibid., 292). In practice, the term "operational feasibility" is thus used as if a project that works in one relatively resource-poor country, such as Brazil, should work in all poor countries—as if differences in context are insignificant. Operational feasibility, as it is currently conceived, does not adequately take account of political barriers to the successful implementation of global health projects. It would be worthwhile to let operational feasibility refer primarily to logistics and to deal with other barriers to eradication under another rubric.

## *The Importance of Politics*

The resistance that I believe hobbles the Polio Eradication Initiative is intimately tied to politics. Within a district, the behaviors I believe form a matrix of resistance are intensely political in at least two senses. First, what goes on at the district level is deeply shaped by "office politics," usefully defined as "the management of influence to obtain ends not sanctioned by the organization or to obtain sanctioned ends through non-sanctioned influence means" (Mayes and Allen 1977, 675). Patron-clientism, falsification, and corruption are examples. They are also forms of resistance.

Second, resistance at the district level is tied to local electoral politics. Were the quality of polio immunization campaigns an election issue in Pakistan, there would be much greater pressure from elected officials on district health leadership to conduct high-quality campaigns. Without such pressure, the influence of electoral politics on the trajectory of polio eradication may be negative, as in the anecdotes I heard about poor-performing workers being retained because an elected official wanted the support of their extended families. In the context of limited or passive public support for a given public health initiative, a district health administration is likely to resist the insistence of international agencies that it take top priority.

At the national level too resistance is political, related both to resentment over agenda setting by powerful nations, and to the myriad other pressing political issues facing the nation's leaders. In a country that often appeared to be sliding toward civil war, it is not likely that Musharraf—facing serious threats to his legitimacy from groups as diverse as the Taliban and lawyer's associations—lost sleep over the incidence of polio cases. The political context in which an eradication program is carried out will affect how much attention high-level government officials can give to it, and how much they may resist the insistence of international officials that the program be a national priority.

Given the importance of politics to the trajectories of eradication programs, it would be useful to introduce a third dimension of feasibility, political feasibility. This would include an analysis of the likelihood that governments would find commitment to a given project compelling from a political, and not simply a humanitarian, point of view. While planners currently spend considerable energy evaluating the impact of political considerations on health projects, their discussions are marred by several conceptual weaknesses. They largely ignore the issue of international power relations, they too readily accept spoken support as actual support, and they incorrectly assume that global health officials can generate political support for a given global health goal.

## Political Considerations in Eradication

One influential framing of the factors necessary to eradicate a disease focuses on "societal and political criteria" for eradication rather than on "operational feasibility." Outlined at the Dahlem Workshop in 1999, it includes these observations:

- The limitations, potential risks, and points of caution for eradication programmes include . . . the potential that programmes will not address national priorities in all countries, and that some countries will not follow the eradication strategy; the perception of programmes as "donor driven."
- Political commitment must be gained at the highest levels, following informed discussion at regional and local levels. A clear commitment of resources from international sources is essential from the start. A resolution by the World Health Assembly is a vital booster to the success of any eradication programme. (Dowdle 1999)

The first point lays out the reasons for the resistance of national and local governments to eradication programs. But the steps proposed to overcome these problems, listed in the second point, have proved insufficient in the Polio Eradication Initiative in Pakistan. While structural power is sufficient to secure spoken support by the Pakistani government for polio eradication—including statements by the highest-level politicians and votes at the World Health Assembly—it is not sufficient to ensure the actual commitment of the government at the levels necessary to secure eradication. The statement that "political commitment must be gained" at all levels is unrealistic. How is one to gain political commitment simultaneously in all areas of all countries in the world for a project that many feel does not address their most urgent needs? As the Pakistani case illustrates, no amount of propaganda is enough when a country has other pressing problems. There are also many relevant aspects of the "political"—wars, coup attempts, elections—over which the actions of global health officials are likely to have little influence.

## *Political Will*

The concept of "political will" is often used in arguments for the importance of government commitment in global health. For example, in 2006, a polio eradication press release mentioned political will as a key factor in the remaining four polio-endemic countries, quoting a senior CDC official: "Eradicating polio is no longer a technical issue alone. Success is now more a question of the political will to ensure effective administration at all levels so that all children get vaccine." Similarly, a representative of Rotary said: "Polio eradication hinges on vaccine supply, community acceptance, funding and political will. The first three are in place. The last will make the difference" (World Health Organization 2006d).

The emphasis on political will is on some level correct. If politicians at all levels in Pakistan suddenly decided that the eradication of polio was their first priority, the virus would not have much of a future there. However, as the anthropologist Lynn Morgan has pointed out, the concept of political will leaves too much out of the picture:

> The international agencies' recent emphasis on "political will" is misguided in three ways. First, "political will" focuses analytic attention on the individual country, thus directing attention away from the crucial role played by the agencies themselves in determining the health policies of less-developed countries. Second, it implies that the political structures within each country are comprised of unified groups that can choose to forge unified national health policy, without considering how internal conflicts may inhibit this process. Third, it implies that health improvements depend simply on commitment by international leaders, thus diverting attention from global relations of dependency and institutionalized inequality that create and perpetuate poverty and ill health in many less-developed countries. (Morgan 1989, 233)

Morgan's critiques hold true for polio eradication in Pakistan, a project that encounters resistance because of its externally mandated nature in a country whose lack of a unified power structure is unquestionably an issue. The concept of political feasibility, then, should address the very real issues that the concept of political will aims to represent, while better taking into account power relations and appreciating the complexity of politics.[9]

Global health's culture of optimism shifts into high gear when it meets a tricky and frustrating issue like a lack of political will. Rather than examine the underlying causes of political problems, the common reaction is to advocate the creation of whatever is lacking—in this case, political will—as if it were a birthday cake that just required the right ingredients. In the quote that opens this chapter, Bill Gates spoke of political will as something it is possible to "generate." In the case of polio eradication in Pakistan, the spoken support of high-level politicians has been generated by the application of structural power, but actual support or will has proved more difficult to come by.[10]

## Evaluating Feasibility

In short, I find three major flaws in most official, on-paper policy about the need for political support for global health initiatives. First, it is too easily assumed that spoken and symbolic support, whether in the form of a vote at the World Health Assembly or a warm reception for a WHO official from Geneva, equals substantive commitment to a given global health goal. In the case of polio eradication, the Pakistani government had little reason not to give the project its spoken support, but it also had many more immediate priorities. Second, the assumption that political will can be created or generated is a facile one. Verbal support is probably possible to generate, given judicious application of power, but actual support is a trickier issue, possible in some cases but not in others. Third, discussions of politics in the global health literature largely ignore the elephant-in-the-room issue of power relations: global health goals are set by the world's rich and powerful, implemented in part with the aid of structural power, and resistance to such power is to be expected.

Evaluating political feasibility should involve an honest evaluation of power relations in the project in question. What are the structures of power in the project? How extensive is the support needed for the project from governments whose actual commitment will likely be minimal? What reasons might these governments have to resist carrying out international mandates (i.e., no great perceived benefit to the politicians in question; large investments of time and energy required)? How much control does a given national government have over local areas within its boundaries?

The answers to these questions can help planners predict where they will likely have problems. Still, by themselves, they are insufficient to predict where difficulties will occur. After all, based on these criteria—little compelling reason to support polio eradication as a priority health strategy, other competing political priorities—many countries should have had problems eliminating polio. Yet it is only in India, Pakistan, Afghanistan, and Nigeria that endemic transmission continues.

This is because epidemiology matters too. Resistance is especially problematic in areas where the elimination of polio is already difficult. In the hot, densely populated cities of India and Pakistan, where sanitation infrastructure may consist only of an open sewer, poliovirus transmission is the world's most intense. Also, as I discussed in Chapter 2, the oral polio vaccine is less effective in these areas. Here, campaign quality must be near perfect if elimination is to be achieved: the margin of error is so thin that resistance can easily sustain polio transmission. In places where the task was easier—because of lower population density, a cooler climate, better vaccine efficacy, better sanitation infrastructure, or freedom from instability and unrest—the task of eliminating polio was achievable even where resistance was present.

Take, for example, Pakistan's mountainous Northern Areas and Azad Kashmir. In these areas, cities and villages are tucked among the peaks of the Karakorams and Himalayas. There, I worked in a city where indicators of campaign quality were among Pakistan's worst. Yet there has been no polio transmission in that area since 2000; a lower population density and a cold climate made the elimination of poliovirus relatively easy. Resistance was a problem there. I went to trainings where not a single person showed up; teams skipped days of work; the street-level plans, so meticulously prepared in Kaifabad, were in disarray. Still, polio transmission had been halted, and not a single case had been found in six years.

In places where eliminating a given disease is politically difficult but epidemiologically relatively easy, then, eradication programs might still make rapid progress. The converse is also true: in areas that are epidemiologically difficult but where political commitment is forthcoming, elimination may be relatively straightforward.

China provides an interesting case study of this second type. Concerned about an epidemic of polio that struck in 1989–1990, the Chinese government started regional immunization campaigns in 1990, and carried out six national campaigns in 1993–1995. These campaigns were stunningly effective: by 1995 or soon thereafter, endemic poliovirus circulation within China had ceased (Centers for Disease Control and Prevention 1994; Chiba et al. 1992; Hoekstra et al. 2000; Ke-an et al. 1997; Yang et al. 1995).

Part of the reason for the dramatic success of the Chinese campaigns is that they were carried out with the full commitment of a relatively cohesive and powerful government. China paid for over 90 percent of the costs of the campaigns itself, and it was able to coordinate Ministry of Health activities with mass media and local governments. More than 80 million children were immunized in the initial national campaigns; about a third of the children under one had not been previously immunized (Jian et al. 1998; Ke-an et al. 1997; World Health Organization 1997; Yang et al. 1995).

The project of polio elimination in China, while challenging—high population density and poverty were undeniable factors in ongoing polio circulation—was still somewhat easier than in Pakistan (Yang et al. 1995). Across much of China, the climate is sufficiently cold that the heat-sensitive vaccine could be carried for days without ice packs and still retain efficacy (World Health Organization 1997). The country had a strong network of primary health care, and relatively high rates of routine immunization had already pushed polio into decline (Ward and Hull 1995). In part because of these factors, elimination was achieved despite surveillance that was not as strong as Pakistan's is now, and despite the fact that immunization coverage in mobile populations was less than 50 percent in one study (Chiba et al. 2001; Nakano et al. 1997; Zhang et al. 1997). Still, government commitment was a significant factor in the rapid elimination of polio from China. One man I talked to who had worked on immunization campaigns in both China and Pakistan said the difference was striking—in contrast with Pakistan, he said, "once the government of China decides to do something, they *do* it."

Pakistan is a case of difficult epidemiology *overlapping* with resistance to cause difficulties. Elimination of polio from Pakistan is epidemiologically harder than in China: high population density, hot climate, and poor sanitation infrastructure lead to intense virus transmission that is difficult to interrupt. Poor security, too, presents significant challenges. Still, as I mentioned in Chapter 5, polio transmission was interrupted in the Punjab—probably the most epidemiologically difficult area of Pakistan—for several years. So resistance is an important factor as well.

The analysis of political feasibility in an eradication program, then, should overlap with existing analyses of technical and operational feasibility. Each of these analyses should be fine-grained. Technical and political feasibility should not be assessed in a global sense until they have been mapped. Such mapping is critical because it is in areas where epidemiological and political difficulties overlap that elimination of a given disease will be a challenge. In epidemiologically easy areas, resistance may not form a major obstacle to the elimination of a disease like polio. In areas where both epidemiology and politics present challenges, difficulties in elimination are likely. In such areas, alternative strategies to secure eradication should be prepared ahead of time.

## Planning for Flexibility

The major block polio eradication faces is that planners and officials know of problems but can do little about them. The World Health Organization is an organization of governments, with its policy set, at least officially, by the World Health Assembly, a forum in which each country has one vote. WHO employees' official role is to advise and assist governments in doing whatever they have decided to do. While this is not how things may work in practice, the fiction of government ownership ties the hands of WHO officials. As an organization of governments, the WHO cannot bypass those governments.

The spearheading partners in the Polio Eradication Initiative have a division of labor that fits each organization's strengths and generally works quite well. The American CDC assists with technical advice and the creation of world-class laboratories across the world. UNICEF focuses on social mobilization. And the World Health Organization runs the surveillance system and is responsible for oversight of vaccination campaigns.

Over twenty years, these roles have become so institutionally entrenched that I never heard the possibility of changing them discussed. In these end-stages of the project, what would be strengths in most times and places have become weaknesses. The World Health Organization, with access to every country in the world and an extensive staff trained in epidemiology and public health, would seem an ideal organization to oversee a worldwide eradication project. But when it meets with government resistance, it is helpless. It cannot circumvent the government.[11]

Conceptualizing the problems that polio eradication is facing as "resistance" makes the World Health Organization's difficulty clear and points the way to a different course of action. The Polio Eradication Initiative is a vast partnership with many diverse stakeholders. This could be a strong asset in times of trouble if flexibility—the option to draw on the varied strengths of the organizations involved—had been built into the system from the start.

In polio eradication, in large measure, all the agencies involved have accepted the World Health Organization's structural limitations as the Polio Eradication Initiative's structural limitations. An eradication program demands the opposite: that everyone involved use every last bit of influence they have in the endgame. Although the World Health Organization has to work only through governments, not all the partners in a major eradication program are so limited. In the case of polio eradication, major donors and partners like Rotary International and USAID could work with other sorts of agencies—NGOs, local village leadership, or religious organizations, to name a few.

The eradication programs of the future will also be partnerships. The potential flexibility of an initiative with a diversity of organizations involved is a powerful and currently untapped resource. What is needed is planned adaptability, alternate strategies folded into the system from the start. Here, I outline what such a plan might have looked like in the case of polio eradication.

## A Flexible Structure

The ultimate success of smallpox eradication was due in part to institutional flexibility. In that project, planners were flexible enough to switch from the method of mass vaccination to the controversial but ultimately more effective technique of surveillance and containment, securing eradication. In the case of polio, because of the nature of the virus and the vaccine, mass vaccination is the only method available. But while there are limits on methodological flexibility in polio eradication, more structural and organizational flexibility are possible.

As the elimination of polio from most of the world illustrates, the current organizational system for polio eradication is in most places a good one. However, continued transmission in four countries indicates that this system is not ideal everywhere. What is needed in polio eradication is a way to create new organizational structures in areas where the standard protocol is not working.

A framework for creating such structures could have been built into the project. Polio eradication had several deadlines for securing eradication: first, 2000 (entirely unrealistic given the project's late scale-up) and subsequently, 2005 (which gave countries like Pakistan the time they required). Missing the second deadline could have served as a watershed moment for the project, a time for changing strategies and reorganizing structures that were not working. The Polio Eradication Initiative's partner agencies could have agreed *ahead of time* that missing the 2005 deadline would be a sign that structural changes were necessary. The creation of these contingency plans could take place over the several years before the deadline, so that the program would experience neither delay nor interruption. What follows is a possible framework for such changes.

The existing structure would remain the same in districts where transmission had been interrupted for some significant length of time, perhaps a year.[12] This would consolidate the considerable gains the Polio Eradication Initiative had made and allow institutional memory to remain intact in areas where the system functioned fairly well.

In districts where polio remained stubbornly entrenched, the structure of implementation (though not the basic methods) would change entirely. The World Health Organization would no longer be responsible for overseeing campaigns in those areas. Instead, a partner that could work with agencies *outside* governments would take on that responsibility. There would be several key advantages in bypassing the government in difficult districts. First, the leadership of the new partner organization in question would have more choice about whether to take on polio eradication than the district government did, and hence could reasonably be expected to be more committed to that goal. Second, there could be *direct* lines of accountability and control between the Polio Eradication Initiative and a local NGO in ways not possible between the World Health Organization and a district government.

The World Health Organization, then, would cede its role to another partner in problematic districts. The choice of agency would depend on the area in question; Rotary International, while not currently involved in administration of polio eradication activities in a major way, is one possibility. Alternately, USAID, which routinely implements projects in Pakistan in partnership with NGOs as well as the government, might be able to administer campaigns in some areas.[13] (While USAID is not an official spearheading partner, it is a major donor and currently involved in funding vaccine procurement and social mobilization for polio eradication in Pakistan.) Polio eradication leadership could also look beyond the usual suspects in implementing agencies to consider atypical and perhaps more productive partners in particularly tough areas. For example, the government of Saudi Arabia has contributed to polio eradication and might be able to forge unconventional partnerships in security-compromised areas. None of the agencies mentioned here have agreed to take on such roles thus far. This is less a roadmap than some suggestions and a call for flexibility and creativity in looking for agencies that would work in difficult areas.

Such an international overseeing agency would probably need to hire an implementing organization in the district in question, and again unconventional choices should be considered. While health NGOs would be obvious choices, they do not exist in all places nor would they always be the best at implementing vaccination campaigns. The beauty of polio immunization is that it requires almost no health knowledge to carry out effectively. Religious organizations, local groups, or NGOs from other sectors might be possible implementing agencies.

NGOs or other organizations would likely not be free of some of the same problems that exist in government health systems. Patron-clientism is certainly present in NGOs in South Asia (Lewis 2004). Dissatisfaction over the poor pay provided to ground-level female workers would not disappear just because the agency providing employment was an NGO rather than the government (cf. Sharma 2006). Nonetheless, the involvement of NGOs in areas of particular challenge would create direct lines of accountability impossible in the current system.

In designing district-level backup plans, contracting with agencies that have significant ties to the communities they will need to reach is a worthwhile goal. Agencies should have support and legitimacy in the populations they will be serving. However, it should be accepted that polio immunization is not, and will not become, a major priority for recipient populations in Pakistan. Thus, the expectations for contributions from local populations should be kept realistic. Contracting agencies, for example, cannot reasonably be expected to carry out repeated, time-intensive immunization campaigns with volunteer labor.

## Planning Ahead

Planning for which NGOs or other organizations could be alternate agencies should take place on a district-by-district basis, and in some cases on levels below that of the district. The first step, taken several years before alternate agencies would need to take over, would be studies (perhaps ethnographic studies) of organizations with the reach and motivation to carry out such a major project in the problematic districts.

Early planning is essential to avoid the calcification of roles that currently characterizes polio eradication. The basic design of the backup plan for polio eradication would need to be negotiated with the government well ahead of the target date for eradication. This negotiation might prove difficult, or it might be a relief to government officials to have an alternate strategy in the wings for which they do not shoulder so much responsibility and so much blame. Also, as the potential embarrassment of being relieved of polio eradication duties would fall primarily to district governments, the national government might be willing to agree to such a proposal. Ultimately, if the structural power of international organizations is sufficient to drive policy to the extent that eradication programs with no overwhelming local support can become national priorities, that same structural power can be used to dictate the terms of implementation of these eradication programs.

Microlevel planning is key to the success of backup plans. No organization save the national government will likely be large enough to take over operations for an entire country, nor should it; in areas where the government is doing a good job, it would be unwise to replace it. Other large organizations that might be excellent agencies for certain areas of the country—the example of the extraordinarily well-organized and well-received Aga Khan Health Services in Pakistan's Northern Areas leaps to mind—would be liabilities in other areas. The Aga Khan Health Services, in this example, serves primarily Ismaili Muslims, a minority group; it does not have a large infrastructure and staff or widespread popular trust and support in most parts of the country.

In some districts, particularly in urban districts with huge populations, the problem of districtwide coverage might be tackled most effectively by having several organizations cover different areas of the district. Each agency should focus on areas where they are strong. As long as the boundaries each agency serves are clear—something which should be fairly simple given the street-by-street maps and plans that the Polio Eradication Initiative has already generated—such division might allow each agency to serve areas where they are most likely to be well informed and well received. Monitors from a given agency could also be dispatched to assess the coverage rates of another agency, which might lead to more accurate feedback on problem areas.

Planning and training of the organizations chosen as backup agencies would need to start about a year before they took over. This would give them time to get up to speed in terms of the planning and organization needed to carry out such a major project. World Health Organization personnel that know a lot about the areas in question could be transferred to the implementing agency to create some institutional knowledge and memory.[14]

Shifting to a new and untried strategy of course carries risks. However, repeating the things that have not worked in the past is an excellent recipe for failure. While shifting the responsibility for campaigns to a different set of organizations would represent a huge change, not *all* polio eradication activities in troubled districts need be changed. Activities that the government agencies and WHO are handling well on their own—such as surveillance in Pakistan—should be left the way they are. Having different agencies carrying out immunization campaigns and surveillance could improve surveillance accuracy, since the discovery of cases would no longer reflect poorly on the district government reporting them. These suggestions are for the *end-stages* of an eradication program only, for those last few intractable areas. Shifting control to local agencies would be complicated, chaotic, and likely ineffective if attempted on a widespread basis too early in such a project.

It is probably too late for polio eradication to become flexible; such plans likely could not be implemented now. But it is not too late for other eradication programs to think very hard about ways that they could be flexible in areas where eradication proves difficult. The strategy I outline here for polio eradication might transfer fairly well to a measles eradication program. It is hard to know exactly how these suggestions might apply to a malaria eradication project, since the tools to eradicate malaria do not currently exist.

I am wary of being seduced by the culture of optimism myself, of falling into the trap of presenting a tweak that would secure eradication. The strategy I suggest here is not a cure or a panacea for the variety of very tough obstacles that eradication programs face. But explicit awareness of power relationships and resistance as well as formal planning for institutional flexibility would, I believe, better position eradication programs to reach their goals. Taking these steps might shift the balance from the possible toward the probable.

# Notes

## CHAPTER 1

1.  More information on the history and progress of the Polio Eradication Initiative is in Chapter 2.
2.  The World Health Organization valued employees who were aware of local realities. At all levels of the organization, there was an emphasis on understanding the particularities of specific situations—the motto in Pakistan for 2007 was "local solutions to local problems." Perhaps five decades of anthropological harping on this point has had an impact.
3.  Most of the conversation quoted in this chapter took place in Urdu, or in a local dialect of Punjabi. (In this particular case, the exchange took place in a mixture of Urdu and English.) The translations into English are my own. Throughout the book, speech in quotation marks or in block quotes (such as this one) represents either a direct quote recorded at the time or a conversation reconstructed immediately after it took place.
4.  Minority groups across Pakistan and India were consistently less well vaccinated than the general population. This was in many cases due to prejudice on the part of the lower-middle-class, mainstream-culture vaccinators, an issue I discuss in more detail in Chapter 5.
5.  District-level health staff were supposed to carry out a variety of tasks for "social mobilization," including visiting teachers and religious and community leaders on a regular basis to secure their support for immunization activities. Overall, refusals were a concern but not a major barrier to the elimination of polio from Pakistan; by the WHO's best estimates, they never amounted to more than 1 percent of the overall population.
6.  The Global Alliance for Vaccines and Immunizations (GAVI); the Global Fund to Fight AIDS, Tuberculosis, and Malaria; the Stop TB Partnership; and the Measles Initiative are notable examples of large projects similar in these respects to the Polio Eradication Initiative. The projects are of course not exactly alike—the Global Fund, for example, uses a much wider array of implementing organizations in recipient countries than the Polio Eradication Initiative does—but my discussion of the challenges that the Polio Eradication Initiative faces likely applies to some extent to these other large projects.

7.  I am aware that what, exactly, constitutes success and failure is often a deceptively simple question. David Mosse argues that in some projects, attribution of "success" or "failure" depends less on what actually happens on the ground than on whether planners are able to cast the achievements of a project in terms of their donors' dominant paradigms (Mosse 2005). In the culture of optimism that I argue characterizes global health, projects that are failures by their original criteria may be recast as successes (Brown 1998). Also, projects that succeed in their stated goals may have few wider impacts (the eradication of polio, for example, would not significantly change the overall burden of disease in Pakistan). These nuances must be grappled with—but discussing them should assist with, rather than detract from, the goal of analyzing whether and how development projects are making concrete improvements in the lives of the poor they aim to assist.

8.  The Polio Eradication Initiative does a genetic sequence of the poliovirus obtained from every child with polio, which enables analysis of the patterns of transmission of the virus.

9.  Eight to ten million people fled in both directions across these newly drawn lines in the Punjab and Bengal, and between half a million and a million people were killed (Menon and Bhasin 1998, 35). Bangladesh, formerly East Pakistan, became an independent nation after a civil war in 1971.

10. The government estimated that as of 2000–2001, 32 percent of the population was surviving on less than Rs 748 (about $13) per person per *month*, the poverty threshold "derived by valuing the minimum required caloric intake of 2350 calories per capita with a minimum expenditure required for non-food needs" (Government of Pakistan Planning Commission 2005, 7). It should be noted that the economic situation in Pakistan as a whole has improved since this estimate was made in 2000.

11. I attended a lower-middle-class wedding within earshot of the bombs exploding at Lal Masjid during the "operation," and conversation at the wedding centered on this topic. While there was widespread condemnation of the actions of the militants—most people felt that their using the children of the madrassah as a human shield was reprehensible, and that their lack of respect for private property was a serious problem—the actions of the government were also widely criticized. Why had the government allowed the militants to get so strong and then gone in with military force, instead of using more subtle tactics from the beginning, like disconnecting the electricity and water in the mosque? The deaths of the children inside the mosque (nobody trusted the government's assurances that only a few children remained inside) were certainly the government's responsibility as well. Probably, people speculated, Musharraf was under pressure from the United States to look tough on terror.

12. Throughout this book, Urdu transliterations follow Platts's *Dictionary of Urdu, Classical Hindi, and English* (Platts 2004).

13. Numbers of children under five reported immunized to the Polio Eradication Initiative were as high as 20 percent of these overall population numbers in some districts. Pakistan does have a very young population overall, and there is probably some inflation by district health staff of the numbers of children immunized, but the census figures quoted here are likely underestimates of the actual population.

14. Lady health workers are part-time employees of the government health department whose job is to provide basic health information to other families in their communities. They also go door-to-door vaccinating children during polio campaigns. Their role is discussed in more detail later in the book.

15. My position on this matter has been influenced by writers in the so-called "reflexive turn" in anthropology, as well as by feminist critiques of science, especially the (slightly differing) viewpoints of Sandra Harding, Donna Haraway, and Evelyn Fox Keller (Haraway 1988; Harding 1991, 2004; Keller 1985; Keller and Longino 1996). Lila Abu-Lughod does a nice job tying these literatures together in her piece "Can There Be a Feminist Ethnography?" (Abu-Lughod 1990a).

16. In northern Nigeria, there has been fairly widespread popular opposition to polio vaccination (Jegede 2007; Pallansch and Sandhu 2006; Renne 2006); this is not the case in Pakistan, where refusals appear to make up less than 1 percent of the population.

## CHAPTER 2

1. The epigraph sources, in order, are: Thigpen 2004; Boyd 2007; and Chan 2007b.

2. The definition of the term "eradication" is the subject of some debate (Miller, Barrett, and Henderson 2006; World Health Organization 1998b). The definition I use here was established at the Dahlem Workshop (Dowdle 1999).

3. The definition of "elimination" I use in this book is the one established at the Dahlem Workshop (Dowdle 1999). It is the definition used in eradication programs, including polio eradication. "Elimination" may mean different things in other disease-control programs, for example, in the case of leprosy, "elimination" has been defined as reducing the prevalence of disease to less than one case per ten thousand people (Lockwood and Suneetha 2005). This is not elimination in the sense I use the term here, as transmission is ongoing.

4. As the project was not yet global, the goal would be described as "elimination" in today's terms.

5. Many people in the South at that time did not have privies (Ettling 1981).

6. The International Health Division's name changed several times; it was also called the International Health Commission and the International Health Board. Here, I use International Health Division to refer to all of these entities to avoid confusion.

7. The 1958 World Health Assembly, where the Soviets argued in favor of smallpox eradication, was the first that the USSR had attended in about a decade. Although enthusiasm for yet another eradication program was not forthcoming, WHO's member countries for diplomatic reasons unanimously approved the proposal to eradicate smallpox (Tucker 2001).

8. The method that was adopted, case detection and containment, is described in more detail in Chapter 6. Because of the epidemiology of polio transmission, it is not a feasible strategy in polio eradication.

9. As in the case of polio eradication, discussed later, the Dracunculiasis [guinea worm] Eradication Program has consistently instituted optimistic target dates

for eradication. Initially, the program aimed to eradicate guinea worm by 1995 (Tayeh and Cairncross 2007).

10. In the case of polio, vaccination will need to be continued even after eradication because of ongoing circulation of vaccine viruses that could become virulent; however, it is hoped that at some point polio vaccination could cease entirely (World Health Organization 2006a).

11. Similarly, workers in the Smallpox Eradication Program had, in the words of one observer, "messianic impulses" (Greenough 1995, 644). In the interests of making potential biases clear, I note that I am agnostic in respect to eradication.

12. While Vitamin A supplementation and, in limited areas, other basic health interventions have been integrated with polio campaigns, they are not the focus of the campaigns and certainly do not constitute comprehensive health care. Because only three or four doses of oral polio vaccine are administered during routine immunizations, and many children in areas with poor sanitation and high temperatures require as many as ten doses of vaccine before they are immune to polio (Grassly et al. 2007), even routine immunization coverage of 100 percent might not halt transmission of the disease entirely in places like Northern India.

13. Mass vaccination campaigns against polio had been carried out in Brazil before, in the 1970s, but not in a coordinated way across the entire country (Risi 1997).

14. A number of industrialized countries, including the United States, England, Japan, Czechoslovakia, and sections of the Soviet Union, had also achieved elimination of polio using mass campaigns.

15. Unlike current polio campaigns in much of the world, which deliver OPV door-to-door, in Brazil parents had to bring their children to a fixed site to receive polio vaccine. In the Americas, it was only at the very last stages of the program that house-to-house "mop-up" campaigns were carried out, and then only in less than 10 percent of districts in Latin America and the Caribbean (de Quadros 1997a).

16. Unlike WHO, UNICEF was enthusiastic about vertical programs (Muraskin 1998).

17. Rotary's choice of polio as the disease to be targeted was influenced by Rotarian John Sever, who had ties to Albert Sabin and was chief of infectious disease at the National Institutes of Health (Pigman 2005).

18. Until this time, Rotary had legislation that *prevented* nationally or internationally coordinated service projects: in 1923, it had adopted a resolution stating that each Rotary club should choose its own projects and that Rotary International (the governing body of the organization) "should never prescribe nor proscribe any objective activity for any club" (Pigman 2005, 18).

19. Sabin, having developed the oral polio vaccine, spent many years advocating for polio eradication, and his celebrity advanced the project, but he could at times be a difficult person to work with (Hampton 2009).

20. According to Herbert Pigman, involved in leading Rotary's PolioPlus program in these years: "Health officials were wary of Rotary, an organization with no significant experience in public health affairs. . . . Rotary's financial pledge to buy oral polio vaccine, however, was too good to ignore" (Pigman 2005, 76–77).

21. Rotarian Herbert Pigman writes that Rotary's addition of the "plus" to PolioPlus was a response to WHO's concerns about vertical programs, "a compromise strategy faithful to [Rotary's] own dream of polio eradication yet supportive of broader immunization goals" (Pigman 2005, 34).

22. Whether or not this has actually been the case—whether polio eradication has strengthened or detracted from routine immunization coverage worldwide—is a hotly contested issue discussed in more detail in Chapter 5.

23. Although for limited periods of time in certain areas, other strategies have been attempted (for example, India experimented with immunizing children under three), immunizing children under five has nearly always been the strategy used. Oral polio vaccine is preferred to injectable polio vaccine for mass campaigns because it is cheaper and can be administered by workers with minimal training.

24. Pakistan carried out its first campaign in 1994, but India did not begin eradication activities until 1996.

25. Because surveillance in China was somewhat weak at that time, the exact date of elimination is unclear, but elimination was achieved.

26. Rotary had begun lobbying the U.S. government in 1994, a new activity for the organization and one that was "foreign to its traditions" (Pigman 2005, 85). The effort was effective; Rotary could raise much more money for polio eradication through lobbying than it could through its membership alone.

27. The reason for the lower efficacy of oral polio vaccine in places like India is likely that the same factors that make poliovirus highly prevalent in these areas—a warm climate, high population density, and poor sanitation—are also favorable conditions for a range of enteroviruses that compete with vaccine virus in a child's gut. They may keep the vaccine virus from infecting the child (and triggering the immune response that would make the child immune to paralytic wild polio). In addition, diarrhea in children, common in these areas, may flush the vaccine virus out of the child's system before it has a chance to infect the child. Finally, high levels of maternal antibodies against polio in young infants may affect vaccine efficacy (Grassly et al. 2006; Hull et al. 1994).

28. As I discuss in more detail later, the new vaccines have their own drawbacks. Specifically, they confer immunity to only one of the two types of currently circulating poliovirus.

29. Surveillance data for Pakistan, here and elsewhere in this book, were obtained directly from the National Surveillance Cell in Islamabad.

30. "Wild" is the term used to describe naturally circulating poliovirus, as opposed to the form of poliovirus used in the oral polio vaccine.

31. Oral polio vaccine is composed of weakened live poliovirus, which can be transmitted between individuals. In general, this is an advantage of OPV, as it means that people who never received the vaccine themselves can be "vaccinated" secondhand by contracting vaccine virus from vaccinated contacts. However, in the rare cases when the weakened vaccine virus evolves into a virulent form, its transmissibility becomes a liability. Injectable polio vaccine, the type currently used in the United States, contains a killed poliovirus and thus does not carry this risk. However, the higher cost of injectable vaccine, and the fact that it must be administered by skilled workers, make it impractical for use in global mass campaigns.

32. "Concentration," here, is number of WHO workers per number of people in the country.

## CHAPTER 3

1. Names and, in a few cases, identifying information of most of the people described in this chapter have been changed.
2. "Teams" was the common appellation for workers doing vaccination, as they always worked in pairs.
3. In some cases, trainees received fifty cents per person from UNICEF for attending trainings, but this was not always the case, and regardless, most people concluded that spending half their day at training was not worth the money. Procuring the money, which was supposed to be for "refreshments," from UNICEF was a constant source of frustration. At the heart of the problem was that UNICEF did not provide the money until after the campaign was over, and determining which area in charges had actually provided refreshments (and thus should be reimbursed themselves) and which had not (in which case the workers should be given the money) was nearly impossible. The two dollars a day workers received during the campaigns was from WHO, and while there was widespread dissatisfaction with the amount, I never heard of problems with its delivery to workers.
4. Each vial of vaccine has a heat-sensitive sticker that changes color if the vaccine is exposed to heat and is thus in danger of losing potency. The "cold chain" that kept vaccine cold as it progressed from its delivery at Islamabad's airport to the farthest reaches of Pakistan's deserts was effective and impressive, a minor marvel of organization and planning.
5. Exclusive schools catering to the wealthiest families in Pakistan were among the most common sites where vaccination was refused.
6. Of the 100 children in my sample of mobile families in and around Kaifabad, only 77 had received oral polio vaccine during the last campaign. Of the 23 children who remained unvaccinated, 19 were missed because no team ever visited their home. Three were missed because the children were unavailable when the team visited, and the team never returned to find them. There was only one child in the sample whose parents refused polio vaccine, on the grounds that the child was, at three months, too young to be vaccinated. It is worth noting that *routine* immunization coverage of standard childhood immunization was very low in this sample of nomads: only 24 percent of children under five had received the full course of routine immunizations. Many mothers mentioned to me that they did not know where to obtain such immunizations.
7. I suggested oral rehydration therapy, a simple, cheap, lifesaving intervention for diarrhea available for pennies within a few blocks of this settlement. The parents already knew about ORT and had been giving their daughter the most expensive, premixed variety—perhaps not a bad idea given the questionable quality of the water available to them.
8. The Polio Eradication Initiative has mapped out the entire country of Pakistan in detail. After more than five years of house-to-house campaigns, even the

number of children under five on each street is known. This is an incredible achievement in a country where no maps of most areas are publicly available.

9. Since the time of my work in Pakistan, the rules have changed: supervisors now count children as missed or covered based on whether their fingers are marked with permanent marker, not on parental report.

## CHAPTER 4

1. As the function of patron-client relationships in this context was primarily to provide job security, and not other material benefits, to the client, they differ from what Weingrod has called "party-patronage" relationships (Weingrod 1968, 381). In such relationships, described in the context of a government health bureaucracy by Dan Smith (Smith 2003), clients receive access to perks such as high-paying contracts in return for political support of a patron. This was emphatically *not* the case in the Polio Eradication Initiative, where little of value to clients was in play; polio vaccine was not a valuable commodity in Pakistan, and pay given for work on polio was much too low for assignment to polio work to be a reward. On the contrary, assignment to polio work was, as for the area in charge discussed earlier, often a dangerous liability: it carried the risk of being fired, with little monetary benefit. It was to protect themselves from this risk of job loss that low-level employees in the Pakistani government health system engaged in patron-client relationships.

2. This ambivalence resembles that of others in poor countries who rely on "corrupt" practices even as they decry them as immoral (Smith 2007).

3. Even this definition, however, presents problems. Poorly paid officials who engaged in such activities often justified them, rightly or not, as getting what was due them from an extraordinarily moneyed project. Foreign consultants enjoyed salaries many orders of magnitude larger than the tiny amounts of money low-level employees were able to pilfer.

4. While I reported this information, no action was ever taken, perhaps because the man in question had successfully established patron-client relationships with influential superiors. I never saw any such instances of pilfering in Kaifabad, a much more tightly run district.

5. This was an ongoing sore point; districts claimed that the census had been of poor quality (which was probably true), and the census did not record the large numbers of Afghan refugees. Nonetheless, as census numbers of children under five were generally divergent from numbers that districts claimed they vaccinated, and as the census numbers were nearly always lower, falsification at one or more levels was probably fairly widespread.

6. James C. Scott notes that "the theatrical imperatives that normally prevail in situations of domination produce a public transcript in close conformity with how the dominant group would wish to have things appear. . . . In the short run, it is in the interest of the subordinate to produce a more or less credible performance, speaking the lines and making the gestures he knows are expected of him" (Scott 1990, 4). In this instance, the international agencies like WHO and UNICEF running polio eradication controlled the public transcript. I discuss the public transcript and power relations further in Chapter 5.

7. Foreign volunteers, unlike their underpaid Pakistani counterparts,

enjoyed a very generous per diem and stayed in some of the country's best accommodations.

8.  What, exactly, constitutes "development" is a can of worms that I probably need not open here. For my purposes here, "development" can be defined as "the successful implementation of development projects." Whether the successful implementation of such programs will lead to "development" in some larger sense is a separate question to which I believe the answer is probably no.

9.  When, in 1996, Pakistan was reported by Transparency International to be the second-most-corrupt state in the world, it was joked that "it was Pakistan's fate never to be first in anything" (Verkaaik 2001, 355).

10. Whether a particular action is "corrupt" is a question that will often be answered differently depending on the position of the person making the determination (Gupta 1995).

11. An awareness of how history shapes patterns of corruption is important. As Scott notes: "Colonial office until the twentieth century was regarded more often than not as an investment in an exclusive franchise that was expected to yield a good return to the political entrepreneur who acquired it" (Scott 1969, 315).

12. Many WHO officials in Islamabad felt strongly that pay for ground-level workers should be raised. Their requests for higher pay for workers were resisted by their superiors in Cairo on the grounds that raising pay for all of Pakistan's 200,000 ground-level workers was prohibitively expensive—and that there was no evidence that raises would increase the quality of work. During the time of my research, pay for lady health workers and other team members was increased 50 percent, from about $1.30 a day to about $2 a day. The lady health workers I spoke to were universally appreciative of this—it was an important gesture materially and symbolically—but felt that pay was still much too low.

13. EPI stands for the Expanded Program on Immunization, the course of routine immunizations given children during the first year of life.

14. Transfers may result in the provincial government giving the EDO in question a "posting for punishment" in a notoriously tough district. Polio eradication officials frequently decried this practice, as it resulted in the worst EDOs being placed in the most difficult districts, compounding problems of management.

15. As Weber pointed out, the introduction of electoral politics into bureaucracies tends to make the bureaucracies less efficient and precise (Weber 1978).

16. These anecdotes were often used to explain why an EDO did not fire a particularly intransigent or poor-performing worker.

17. Musharraf put emphasis on this indicator, and the pay of health post doctors has been raised, so the credit for its improvement may not lie entirely with decentralization, but rural people's ability to demand services from a local elected government is probably not irrelevant.

18. The Polio Eradication Initiative's best estimates of the number of people who refused immunization for their children was less than 1 percent of the total population.

19. I conducted interviews with twenty-six lower-middle-class mothers of children under five in the Punjab. Only one of these women said that she would take her children to the health post if they were missed during polio rounds. The woman in question had adopted a child after ten years of infertility. The child was much

doted on; the mother was exceptional in her unwillingness to expose him to risks of *any* kind.

20. The reasons for the contrast in epidemiology appear to be tied to improved sanitation in wealthy industrialized countries. In places with poor sanitation, the virus is present in the environment at fairly high levels. Most people are infected with the virus at a young age. As infants who contract poliovirus are less likely to become paralyzed than adults, most infants are exposed to "immunizing infections" with poliovirus. (Some of these infants do become paralyzed.) With the development of sanitation infrastructure, infants cease to be infected with poliovirus (and may receive lower levels of maternal antibodies against poliovirus) and thus the natural immunity in a population decreases. This leaves older children and adults susceptible to waves of epidemic, paralytic polio (Smallman-Raynor et al. 2006).

21. About two-thirds of the polio cases reported in 2006 in Pakistan were from the very lowest economic stratum.

22. The term for propaganda in the Polio Eradication Initiative was "social mobilization," which was the explicit responsibility of UNICEF.

23. These workers collected stool samples from everyone in the country under fifteen years old experiencing "acute flaccid paralysis" and sent them to the national lab in Islamabad for testing. As acute flaccid paralysis has many causes other than polio, workers collected and the lab processed samples from more than four thousand cases per year. If poliovirus was found in a stool sample, the virus was genetically sequenced to give information on its relationship to other polioviruses circulating in Pakistan; thus patterns of circulation could be tracked. This was by far the most extensive surveillance system ever developed in Pakistan, and it was reasonably sensitive; while the odd case of polio was almost certainly missed, it is unlikely that the system was blind to significant areas of virus circulation.

24. Highest concentration, here, is per capita population in the country in question. The official name for international consultants was "short-term consultants," the idea being that they were in the country only a brief time, until polio was eradicated. Their contracts were for eleven months. However, in practice many of them stayed in Pakistan for long periods—several for as long as six years.

25. WHO officials would have loved national-level government employees to participate in campaign support in various districts. However, government officials almost never went. The relationship between WHO, UNICEF, and government officials at the national level will be explored in detail in Chapter 5.

26. The situation in the Swat Valley in 2009, where the Taliban placed a moratorium on polio vaccination, is an important exception. However, in all of Pakistan at the time of my research—and in nearly all of the country in 2009—door-to-door polio vaccination campaigns could be carried out, just not always on schedule.

27. This ban and many other security restrictions on mobility UN employees faced were a nearly constant source of friction between UN polio eradication staff and UN security staff. Polio eradication staff largely felt that the security rules were overly restrictive and prevented them from performing their duties in the best possible manner. For example, several foreign consultants got into a heated exchange with a foreign UN security staffer at a meeting over the issue

of the requirement that UN staff ride in four-wheel-drive UN vehicles, usually Land Cruisers, which the polio eradication staff argued were unnecessary and cumbersome in urban areas. The security staff insisted that no concessions could be made on this point.

28. These districts often had a higher percentage of refusals and a low percentage of lady health workers—but, as WHO officials were quick to point out, other districts with these challenges were still able to carry out high-quality campaigns.

## CHAPTER 5

1. Many other global health programs are similarly structured—for example, the Measles Initiative described later in this chapter—despite their status as control, rather than eradication, programs.

2. I do not mean to imply that structural power exists apart from social interaction. Timothy Mitchell suggests that structural power (though he does not use that term) "will seem to be *external* to practice" but is actually "most internal, most integral, and continuously at work *within* social and economic practices" (Mitchell 1990, 571).

3. Farmer here is defining "structural violence," but he means what other theorists refer to as "structural power." While the term "violence" has important uses in Farmer's work, it is not entirely appropriate here. I believe Farmer would agree that while the attempt to deliver polio vaccine multiple times to the most medically underserved children on earth is an endeavor that requires the mobilization of a great deal of power, classifying it as violence would be inaccurate.

4. The weakened live virus in oral polio vaccine can live for years in the guts of immunocompromised individuals, who continue to excrete vaccine virus with the potential to become virulent (Bellmunt et al. 1999). Therefore, immunization cannot cease immediately upon the achievement of eradication. However, it is reasonable to assume that immunization against polio could cease at some point in the future if polio is eradicated.

5. In 2000, the United States switched from oral to injectable polio vaccine, which is generally more expensive but has fewer adverse effects. I was unable to find figures on the amount that the United States now spends per year on injectable polio vaccine, perhaps because it is commonly combined in a single injection with other immunizations.

6. One study analyzing loss of healthy life years (HeaLYs) to various conditions in Pakistan in 1990—before Polio Eradication Initiative activities drastically reduced the polio case count in the country—ranked polio as thirty-fourth among causes of morbidity and mortality in the country. Diarrhea, lower respiratory infections in children, and tuberculosis were the three top contributors to HeaLYs lost (Hyder and Morrow 2000).

7. India and Pakistan were specifically mentioned as countries likely to obstruct the goal of a 90 percent reduction in measles cases globally by 2010 (Centers for Disease Control and Prevention 2007).

8.  Several people suggested that Measles Initiative planners had originally intended to implement measles campaigns only after polio eradication but had decided, when eradication had not been forthcoming, they could not wait any longer to begin work in a country with high measles morbidity and mortality.
9.  An unspoken assumption in this goal was likely that polio would be eradicated before measles activities would be scaled up.
10. Some of the communities in question had organized "demand refusals." Tired of receiving no health services other than polio vaccine, they had attempted to refuse to allow their children to be vaccinated against polio unless other services were also provided. Apparently, the provision of measles vaccine—while far from comprehensive health care—was enough to persuade at least some of these people to accept polio vaccine as well.
11. The per-dose efficacy of mOPV1 against Type 1 paralytic polio was 30 percent in this study, compared to 11 percent for trivalent vaccine (Grassly et al. 2007).
12. For example, WHO estimates of Pakistan's infant mortality rate (80 per 1,000) and its under-five mortality rate (100 per 1,000) are the highest in South Asia, even compared to much poorer countries such as Nepal and Bangladesh (World Health Organization 2007b).
13. The Pakistani army has a reputation for transparency and effectiveness, especially compared to bureaucracies like the Pakistani health system.
14. There are a few notable exceptions in the health sector, such as Edhi (which is best known for providing ambulance services) and the Aga Khan Health Services. While AKHS does provide health services paralleling those of the Pakistani government, it does so only in limited geographical areas.
15. For example, any influence that the Polio Eradication Initiative has on the place of Pakistanis in the world system is insignificant compared to the impact of the war on terror.
16. The lady health worker's response to the pregnant woman was not inappropriate: even if she had wanted to, she could not have assisted with a delivery—even by simply escorting the woman to a health post—and still made her vaccination targets for the day. All the lady health workers' regular tasks, and the tasks of everyone else assigned to polio vaccination, were suspended for the duration of the campaign.
17. The Polio Eradication Initiative carries out genetic sequencing of the poliovirus from each case of polio in Pakistan. That viruses found in different areas of the country are often closely related indicates that mobile populations are transmitting polio from place to place.
18. By the end of 2006, surveillance data indicated that around 95 percent of children aged 0–36 months in Pakistan had received at least three doses of oral polio vaccine.
19. The moratorium on polio vaccination in the Swat Valley in 2009 is an important exception to this generalization. However, the data I am using here are from 2007, prior to that situation—so the conclusion still holds that it is not simply an inability to vaccinate children in security-compromised areas that fosters virus transmission, but the consequences of a lack of supervision in these areas.

## CHAPTER 6

1.  Because I saw different aspects of high-ranking WHO officials' lives in different phases of my fieldwork, Sarah is a composite of several people.
2.  The epigraph quote is from Gates 2008.
3.  Several other cases occurred in 1978 when smallpox virus escaped from a lab in Birmingham, England.
4.  Brilliant first came to India on an overland journey in buses from London to Bangladesh with a "counterculture group" led by Wavy Gravy. Later, he and his wife, inspired by the "LSD saga" of Richard Alpert, returned to India to become devotees of Neem Karoli Baba, a saint with an ashram in the Himalayas. They stayed there until Neem Karoli Baba told Brilliant—who was trained as a doctor—that it was his religious duty to work for the World Health Organization to eradicate smallpox. The WHO was initially skeptical of Brilliant, but he ultimately became part of the core team to organize and lead smallpox eradication in India (Brilliant and Brilliant 1978).
5.  Smallpox was eradicated using the method of case detection and containment, where smallpox cases were actively sought out and quarantined and everyone who had come in contact with the case was vaccinated. Though this method ultimately proved extremely effective at interrupting smallpox transmission, it was initially controversial, as many people felt that mass vaccination of the entire population was a superior strategy.
6.  The official referred to "religious refusal" because the larger discussion was about a few pockets of people who refused vaccination on the grounds that it was unIslamic. In general, Pakistan's most prominent Muslim clerics supported polio immunization.
7.  It is, in other words, the epidemiology of polio itself that rules out search and containment, the strategy used in smallpox eradication, as an effective method in polio eradication.
8.  The vast majority of global public health programs are control programs aimed at keeping transmission of disease low but not at eradicating the disease entirely from the wild. See Chapter 2 for further discussion of the difference between eradication and control.
9.  Eradication programs are special cases. That there is only one successful eradication program to compare with polio eradication weakens my argument here. Certainly, coercive methods alone are not a recipe for success; excellent surveillance, potent vaccines or other tools, and a disease whose epidemiology lends itself to eradication are essential. But in comparing two global eradication programs, one successful and one floundering, one of the key differences that emerges is their method of dealing with resistance.
10. The "window of opportunity" the official was referring to—the elimination of polio from Pakistan by the end of 2007—passed without the goal being met.
11. While I would not yet pronounce polio eradication a failure (perhaps evidence of my own entrapment in the escalation of commitment), the project fits the mold of this literature: it has vastly exceeded original projections of the time and money that would be required to bring it to a successful conclusion.
12. Lionel Tiger refers to this attitude as an "ambient thoughtless optimism which has persisted about economic development" (Tiger 1979, 267).

# CHAPTER 7

1.  The first epigraph is from de Quadros 2004, the second and third from Gates and Gates 2007.
2.  While interruption of transmission has been achieved across the Americas (de Quadros et al. 2004), continuing problems with importation of virus from other parts of the world prevent permanent elimination of the disease from the region (Pan American Health Organization 2009).
3.  With the exception of a few incidents such as vaccine-associated polio outbreaks (e.g., Kew et al. 2002), the Americas have for the most part remained polio free since the elimination of the disease from the region in 1994.
4.  Not surprisingly, many malaria experts view eradication as unattainable. A group of anthropologists who study malaria recently joked that they were planning to title their panel at a major conference "Malaria Eradication: Are You Fucking Kidding Me?"
5.  The parallels between malaria eradication and polio eradication are not perfect. A major reason for the resurgence of malaria was insect resistance to DDT and parasite resistance to chloroquine; biological resistance of this nature is not an issue in polio control because a vaccine is available. However, the disappointment of the failure of malaria eradication also led to malaria's becoming "a low prestige disease, associated with an inglorious past" (Brown 1997, 136). Similar problems would likely arise if the goal of eradication was abandoned in the case of polio.
6.  Speaking later to reporters from the journal *Science*, Chan backpedaled a bit, saying somewhat nonsensically, "It is elimination-slash-eradication, depending on the availability of tools" (Roberts and Enserink 2007, 1544). (See Chapter 2 for the difference between elimination and eradication.)
7.  While those who have been immunized sufficient times will remain immune, children born over the next several years would form a huge underimmunized group more than sufficient to fan transmission. The three doses of oral polio vaccine provided through routine immunizations are not enough to confer immunity in many children, and the WHO's estimates of overall routine immunization coverage, by far the highest estimates I have seen, report around 80 percent of children fully immunized—not enough to seriously limit polio transmission.
8.  The most influential conception of primary health care is the Alma-Ata Declaration, which states: "The people have the right and duty to participate individually and collectively in the planning and implementation of their health care" (World Health Organization 1978, 1).
9.  The use of "political will" to oversimplify complex situations is not unique to practitioners of global health. Political scientist Richard Doner observes that in other segments of the development literature, "political will" is used as a "residual category," sidestepping serious political analysis (Doner 2009, 283).
10. In a few cases, influential politicians have been converted from spoken to actual commitment to the cause by high-level meetings with passionate advocates. Several influential politicians in Pakistan became true polio eradication supporters in this way. However, this strategy does not always work.
11. Even if the World Health Organization is able to get the Ministry of Health on

board for a particular initiative, this does not automatically secure the support of any government as a whole, especially if demands from other sectors such as the military seem more pressing.

12. Determination of whether transmission had actually been interrupted would, of course, have to take the quality of surveillance in the area into account.

13. Anthropologists have criticized the practice of bypassing government health services in favor of NGOs because it weakens the government health system (Pfeiffer 2004). However, in the case of an eradication program, relieving government employees of the responsibility for eradication activities might well free them to do a better job at providing primary health care.

14. Both international and national staff routinely move between the CDC, the WHO, UNICEF, and the Pakistani government, both to take new jobs and to take temporary contracts with the understanding that their old job will await their return. Given this existing fluidity, a mechanism for allowing employees to contract with other agencies on a temporary basis should be possible.

# Works Cited

Abrams, Philip. 1977. Notes on the Difficulty of Studying the State. *Journal of Historical Sociology* 1:58–89.

Abu-Lughod, Lila. 1990a. Can There Be a Feminist Ethnography? *Women and Performance* 5:7–27.

———. 1990b. The Romance of Resistance: Tracing Transformations of Power through Bedouin Women. *American Ethnologist* 17:41–55.

Acharya, Arnab, Jose Luis Diaz-Ortega, Gina Tambini, Ciro de Quadros, and Isao Arita. 2002. Cost-Effectiveness of Measles Elimination in Latin America and the Caribbean: A Prospective Analysis. *Vaccine* 20:3332–3341.

Ahmad, Khabir. 2000. Pakistan Predicts a Polio-Free Future. *Lancet* 356:576.

Arita, I., Miyuki Nakane, and F. Fenner. 2006. Is Polio Eradication Realistic? *Science* 312:852–854.

Asad, Talal. 2004. Where Are the Margins of the State? In *Anthropology in the Margins of the State*, ed. V. Das, D. Poole, 279–288. Santa Fe, N.M.: School of American Research Press.

Asiedu, Kingsley, Bernard Amouzou, Akshay Dharlwal, Marc Karam, Sarat Patnaik, and Andre Meheus. 2008. Yaws Eradication: Past Efforts and Future Perspectives. *Bulletin of the World Health Organization* 86:499–500.

Aylward, R. Bruce, Arnab Acharya, and Sarah England. 2003. Global Health Goals: Lessons from the Worldwide Effort to Eradicate Poliomyelitis. *Lancet* 364:909–914.

Aylward, R. Bruce, Karen A. Hennesey, Nevio Zagaria, Jean-Marc Olive, and Stephen Cochi. 2000. When Is a Disease Eradicable? 100 Years of Lessons Learned. *American Journal of Public Health* 90:1515–1520.

Aylward, R. Bruce, and David L. Heymann. 2005. Can We Capitalize on the Virtues of Vaccines? Insights from the Polio Eradication Initiative. *American Journal of Public Health* 95:773–777.

Aylward, R. Bruce, H. F. Hull, S. L. Cochi, R. W. Sutter, J. M. Olive, and B. Melgaard. 2000. Disease Eradication as a Public Health Strategy: A Case Study of Poliomyelitis Eradication. *Bulletin of the World Health Organization* 78:285–297.

Banta, James E. 2001. From International Health to Global Health. *Journal of Community Health* 26:73–76.

Barrett, Scott. 2004. Eradication versus Control: The Economics of Global Infectious Disease Policies. *WHO Bulletin* 74:35–45.

Barrett, Stanley R. 2002. *Culture Meets Power*. Westport, Conn.: Praeger.

Bart, K. J., J. Foulds, and P. Patriarca. 1996. Global Eradication of Poliomyelitis: Benefit-Cost Analysis. *WHO Bulletin* 74:35–45.

Bate, Roger. 2007. The WHO and Health Targets. *Economic Affairs* 27:102.

Beattie, John. 1964. *Other Cultures*. New York: Free Press.

Bellmunt, Andreas, Gunter May, Roland Zell, Patricia Pring-Akerblom, Willem Verhagen, and Albert Heim. 1999. Evolution of Poliovirus Type I during 5.5 Years of Prolonged Enteral Replication in an Immunodeficient Patient. *Virology* 265:178–184.

Birn, Anne-Emanuelle, and Armando Solorzano. 1999. Public Health Policy Paradoxes: Science and Politics in the Rockefeller Foundation's Hookworm Campaign in Mexico in the 1920s. *Social Science and Medicine* 49:1197–1213.

Boehne, Donna M., and Paul W. Paese. 2000. Deciding Whether to Complete or Terminate an Unfinished Project: A Strong Test of the Project Completion Hypothesis. *Organizational Behavior and Human Decision Processes* 81:178–194.

Boellstorff, Tom. 2008. *Coming of Age in Second Life: An Anthropologist Explores the Virtually Human*. Princeton: Princeton University Press.

Bonu, Sekhar, Manju Rani, and Timothy Baker. 2003. The Impact of the National Polio Immunization Campaign on Levels and Equity in Immunization Coverage: Evidence from Rural North India. *Social Science and Medicine* 57:1807–1819.

Bonu, Sekhar, Manju Rani, and Oliver Razum. 2004. Global Public Health Mandates in a Diverse World: The Polio Eradication Initiative and the Expanded Programme on Immunization in Sub-Saharan Africa and South Asia. *Health Policy* 70:327–345.

Boyd, Bill. 2007. *Ask RI President Bill Boyd. www.rotary.org/interactive/issues/200703/askpresident.html*.

Briggs, Charles, and Clara Mantini-Briggs. 2003. *Stories in the Time of Cholera*. Berkeley: University of California Press.

Brilliant, Lawrence B. 1985. *The Management of Smallpox Eradication in India*. Ann Arbor: University of Michigan Press.

Brilliant, Lawrence B, and Girija Brilliant. 1978. Death for a Killer Disease. *Quest* May/June.

Brockner, Joel. 1992. The Escalation of Commitment to a Failing Course of Action: Toward Theoretical Progress. *Academy of Management Review* 17:39–61.

Brown, Peter J. 1983. Introduction: Anthropology and Disease Control. *Medical Anthropology* 7:1–7.

———. 1997. Culture and the Global Resurgence of Malaria. In *The Anthropology of Infectious Disease*, ed. M. Inhorn, P. J. Brown, 119–141. Amsterdam: Gordon and Breach.

———. 1998. Failure-as-Success: Multiple Meanings of Eradication in the Rockefeller Foundation Sardinia Project, 1946–1951. *Parassitologia* 40:117–130.

Brown, Theodore M., and Elizabeth Fee. 2006. The World Health Organization and the Transition from "International" to "Global" Public Health. *American Journal of Public Health* 96:62–72.

Centers for Disease Control and Prevention. 1993. Recommendations of the International Task Force for Disease Eradication. *Morbidity and Mortality Weekly Report Recommendations and Reports* 42(RR-16): 1–38.

————. 1994. International Notes: Progress toward Poliomyelitis Eradication—
People's Republic of China, 1990–1994. *MMWR* 43:857–859.

————. 2007. Progress in Global Measles Control and Mortality Reduction, 2000–
2006. *Morbidity and Mortality Weekly Report* 56:1237–1241.

Chan, Margaret. 2007a. Urgent Stakeholder Consultation on Interrupting Wild
Poliovirus Transmission. Speech. WHO Headquarters, Geneva. *www.who.int/
dg/speeches/2007/280207_polio/en/index.html.*

————. 2007b. Address by Dr. Margaret Chan, Director-General to the Sixtieth
World Health Assembly. Geneva. *apps.who.int/gb/ebwha/pdf_files/WHA60/
A60_3-en.pdf.*

————. 2007c. Foundation's Vision for Malaria. Comments at the Bill and Melinda
Gates Foundation Malaria Forum. Seattle, Wash. *www.kaisernetwork.org/
health_cast/uploaded_files/101707_malariaforum_part1_transcript.pdf.*

Chandavarkar, Rajnarayan. 1991. Workers' Resistance and the Rationalization of
Work in Bombay between the Wars. In *Contesting Power*, ed. D. Haynes, G.
Prakash, 145–174. Berkeley: University of California Press.

Cheema, Ali, Asim Ijaz Khwaja, and Adnan Qadir. 2005. Decentralization in
Pakistan: Context, Content and Causes. Available at Social Science Research
Network, *ssrn.com/abstract=739712.*

Chiba, Yasuo, Kazuo Hikita, Tsuyoshi Matuba, Tooru Chosa, Shinji Kyoguku,
et al. 2001. Active Surveillance for Acute Flaccid Paralysis in Poliomyelitis
High-Risk Areas in Southern China. *Bulletin of the World Health Organization*
79:103–110.

Chiba, Yasuo, Aiqiang Xu, Li Li, Guifang Liu, Toshiro Takezaki, et al. 1992.
Outbreaks of Paralytic Poliomyelitis and Polio Surveillance in Shandong
Province of China. *Japanese Journal of Medical Science and Biology* 45:255–266.

Childs, Dan. 2007. Despite Advances, Measles Eradication Still Far Off.
*abcnews.go.com/Health/story?id=2808444&page=1.*

Chin, James. 1984. Can Paralytic Poliomyelitis Be Eliminated? *Reviews of Infectious
Diseases* 6:S581–S585.

Coggeshall, L. T. 1944. Anopheles Gambiae in Brazil, 1930–40 (review). *American
Journal of Public Health and the Nations Health* 34:75–76.

Colgrove, James. 2006. *State of Immunity: The Politics of Vaccination in Twentieth-
Century America.* Berkeley: University of California Press.

Cooper, Frederick, and Randall Packard. 2005. The History and Politics
of Development Knowledge. In *The Anthropology of Development and
Globalization*, ed. A. Haugerud, M. Edelman, 126–139. Malden, Mass.:
Blackwell.

Cueto, Marcos. 2004. The Origins of Primary Health Care and Selective Primary
Health Care. *American Journal of Public Health* 94:1864–1874.

Dalrymple, William. 2007. Days of Rage. *New Yorker* 23 July, 26.

Davey, Sheila. 1997. *Polio: The Beginning of the End.* Geneva: World Health
Organization.

de Quadros, Ciro. 1992. Polio Eradication from the Western Hemisphere. *Annual
Review of Public Health* 13:239–252.

————. 1997a. Global Eradication of Poliomyelitis. *International Journal of
Infectious Diseases* 1:125–129.

———. 1997b. Onward towards Victory. In *Polio*, ed. T. M. Daniel, F. C. Robbins, 181–198. Rochester, N.Y.: University of Rochester Press.

———. 2004. Can Measles Be Eradicated Globally? *Bulletin of the World Health Organization* 82:134–138.

de Quadros, Ciro, Jon Kim Andrus, M. Carolina Danovaro-Holliday, and Carlos Castillo-Solorzano. 2008. Feasibility of Global Measles Eradication After Interruption of Transmission in the Americas. *Expert Review of Vaccines* 7:355–362.

de Quadros, Ciro, and D. A. Henderson. 1993. Disease Eradication and Control in the Americas. *Biologicals* 21:335–343.

de Quadros, Ciro, Hector Izurieta, Linda Venczel, and Peter Carrasco. 2004. Measles Eradication in the Americas: Progress to Date. *Journal of Infectious Diseases* 189:S227–S235.

Doner, Richard F. 2009. *The Politics of Uneven Development*. Cambridge: Cambridge University Press.

Donnelly, John. 2007. Goals and Risks Questioned in Polio Eradication Fight. *International Herald Tribune* 22 May.

Dowdle, Walter. 1999. The Principles of Disease Elimination and Eradication. *Morbidity and Mortality Weekly Report* 48:23–27.

Easterley, William. 2006. *The White Man's Burden*. New York: Penguin Press.

Edelman, Marc, and Angelique Haugerud. 2005. Introduction: The Anthropology of Development and Globalization. In *The Anthropology of Development and Globalization*, ed. M. Edelman, A. Haugerud, 1–74. Malden, Mass.: Blackwell.

Elliman, David, and Helen Bedford. 2007. Achieving the Goal for Global Measles Mortality. *Lancet* 369:165–166.

Elyachar, Julia. 2005. *Markets of Dispossession: NGOs, Economic Development, and the State in Cairo*. Durham, N.C.: Duke University Press.

Escobar, Arturo. 1991. Anthropology and the Development Encounter: The Making and Marketing of Development Anthropology. *American Ethnologist* 18:658–682.

———. 1992. Reflections on "Development": Grassroots Approaches and Alternative Politics in the Third World. *Futures* 24:411–436.

———. 1995. *Encountering Development*. Princeton: Princeton University Press.

Ettling, John. 1981. *The Germ of Laziness: Rockefeller Philanthropy and Public Health in the New South*. Cambridge, Mass.: Harvard University Press.

Farley, John. 2004. *To Cast Out Disease: A History of the International Health Division of the Rockefeller Foundation (1913–1951)*. New York: Oxford University Press.

Farmer, Paul. 1992. *AIDS and Accusation*. Berkeley: University of California Press.

———. 1996. Women, Poverty, and AIDS. In *Women, Poverty, and AIDS*, ed. P. Farmer, M. Connors, J. Simmons. Monroe, Maine: Common Courage Press.

———. 1999. *Infections and Inequalities*. Berkeley: University of California Press.

———. 2005. *Pathologies of Power*. Berkeley: University of California Press.

Fenner, F. 1999. Candidate Viral Diseases for Elimination or Eradication. *Morbidity and Mortality Weekly Report* 48:86–90.

Fenner, F., D. A. Henderson, I. Arita, Z. Jezek, and I. D. Ladnyi. 1988. *Smallpox and its Eradication*. Geneva: World Health Organization.

Ferguson, James. 1994. *The Anti-Politics Machine*. Minneapolis: University of Minnesota Press.

————. 2005. Anthropology and Its Evil Twin: "Development" in the Constitution of a Discipline. In *The Anthropology of Development and Globalization*, ed. A. Haugerud, M. Edelman, 140–154. Malden, Mass.: Blackwell.

————. 2006. *Global Shadows*. Durham, N.C.: Duke University Press.

Ferguson, James, and Akhil Gupta. 2002. Spatializing States: Toward an Ethnography of Neoliberal Governmentality. *American Ethnologist* 29:981–1002.

Figueroa, J. P. 1999. Report of the Workgroup on Parasitic Diseases. *Morbidity and Mortality Weekly Report* 48:118–125.

Foege, William. 2005. Preface. In *Global Health Leadership and Management*, ed. W Foege, N. Daulaire, R. E. Black, C. E. Pearson, xv-xxvi. San Francisco: Jossey-Bass.

Foege, William, Nils Daulaire, Robert E. Black, and Clarence E. Pearson, eds. 2005. *Global Health Leadership and Management*. San Francisco: Jossey-Bass.

Foster, George M. 1952. Relationships between Theoretical and Applied Anthropology: A Public Health Program Analysis. *Human Organization* 11:5–16.

————. 1963. The Dyadic Contract in Tzintzuntzan, II: Patron-Client Relationship. *American Anthropologist* 65:1280–1294.

————. 1976. Medical Anthropology and International Health Planning. *Medical Anthropology Newsletter* 7:12–18.

————. 1987. Bureaucratic Aspects of International Health Agencies. *Social Science and Medicine* 25:1039–1048.

Foucault, Michel. 1982. The Subject and Power. *Critical Inquiry* 8:777–795.

Fox, F., and Barry M. Staw. 1979. The Trapped Administrator: The Effects of Job Insecurity and Policy Resistance upon Commitment to a Course of Action. *Administrative Science Quarterly* 24:449–471.

Friedman, Thomas L. 2005. *The World Is Flat*. New York: Farrar, Straus and Giroux.

Garland, Howard, and Donald E. Conlon. 1998. Too Close to Quit: The Role of Project Completion in Maintaining Commitment. *Journal of Applied Social Psychology* 28:2025–2048.

Garrett, Laurie. 2007. The Challenge of Global Health. *Foreign Affairs* January/February, 14–38.

Gates, Bill. 2008. A New Approach to Capitalism in the 21st Century. Speech presented at the World Economic Forum. Davos, Switzerland.

————. 2009. Rotary Polio Speech. *www.rotary.org/RIdocuments/en_pdf/ ia09_gates_speech_en.pdf*.

Gates, Melinda, and Bill Gates. 2007. Foundation's Vision for Malaria. Speeches at the Bill and Melinda Gates Foundation Malaria Forum, Seattle, WA. *www.kaisernetwork.org/health_cast/uploaded_files/101707_malariaforum_part1_ transcript.pdf*.

Government of Pakistan Planning Commission. 2005. Pakistan Millennium Development Goals Report 2005. Islamabad: Centre for Research on Poverty Reduction and Income Distribution. *un.org.pk/undp/publication/PMDGR05.pdf*.

Grassly, Nicholas, Christophe Fraser, Jay Wenger, Jagadish Deshpande, R. W. Sutter, et al. 2006. New Strategies for the Elimination of Polio from India. *Science* 314:1150–1153.

Grassly, Nicholas, Jay Wenger, Sunita Durrani, Sunil Bahl, Jagadish Deshpande, et al. 2007. Protective Efficacy of a Monovalent Oral Type 1 Poliovirus Vaccine: A Case-Control Study. *Lancet* 369:1356–62.

Greenough, Paul. 1995. Intimidation, Coercion and Resistance in the Final Stages of the South Asian Smallpox Eradication Campaign, 1973–1975. *Social Science and Medicine* 41:633–645.

Griffin, Diane, and William Moss. 2006. Can We Eradicate Measles? *Microbe* 1:409–413.

Gubler, D. J. 2004. The Changing Epidemiology of Yellow Fever and Dengue, 1900 to 2003: Full Circle? *Comparative Immunology, Microbiology and Infectious Diseases* 27:319–330.

Gupta, Akhil. 1995. Blurred Boundaries: The Discourse of Corruption, the Culture of Politics, and the Imagined State. *American Ethnologist* 22:375–402.

Gupta, Akhil, and Aradhana Sharma. 2006. Globalization and Postcolonial States. *Current Anthropology* 47:277–307.

Hackett, C. J., and T. Guthe. 1956. Some Important Aspects of Yaws Eradication. *Bulletin of the World Health Organization* 15.

Hahn, Robert. 1999. *Anthropology in Public Health*. New York: Oxford University Press.

Hampton, Lee. 2009. Albert Sabin and the Coalition to Eliminate Polio from the Americas. *American Journal of Public Health* 99:34–44.

Hancock, Graham. 1989. *Lords of Poverty*. New York: Atlantic Monthly Press.

Haraway, Donna. 1988. Situated Knowledges: The Science Question in Feminism and the Privilege of Partial Perspective. *Feminist Studies* 14(3): 575–599.

Harding, Sandra. 1991. *Whose Science? Whose Knowledge?* Ithaca, N.Y.: Cornell University Press.

———, ed. 2004. *The Feminist Standpoint Theory Reader*. New York: Routledge.

Haynes, Douglas, and Gyan Prakash. 1992. Introduction: The Entanglement of Power and Resistance. In *Contesting Power*, ed. D. Haynes, G. Prakash, 1–22. Berkeley: University of California Press.

Henderson, D. A. 1984. The Expanded Programme on Immunization of the World Health Organization. *Reviews of Infectious Diseases* 6:S475–479.

———. 1998. Eradication: Lessons from the Past. *Bulletin of the World Health Organization* 76:17–21.

———. 1999. Lessons from the Eradication Campaigns. *Vaccine* 17:S53-S55.

Hersh, Bradley S., Gina Tambini, Ana Cristina Nogueira, Peter Carrasco, and Ciro de Quadros. 2000. Review of Regional Measles Surveillance Data in the Americas, 1996–99. *Lancet* 355:1943–1948.

Hinman, A. R., W. H. Foege, Ciro de Quadros, P. Patriarca, W. A. Orenstein, and E. W. Brink. 1987. The Case for Global Eradication of Poliomyelitis. *Bulletin of the World Health Organization* 65:835–840.

Hirschman, Albert O. 1967. *Development Projects Observed*. Washington, D.C.: Brookings Institution.

Hoekstra, Edward J., Chai Feng, Wang Xiao-jun, Zhang Xing-lu, Yu Jing-jin, and J. Bilous. 2000. Excluding Polio in Areas of Inadequate Surveillance in the Final Stages of Eradication in China. *Bulletin of the World Health Organization* 78:315–320.

Hoekstra, Edward J., Jeffrey W. McFarland, Catherine Shaw, and Peter Salama.

2006. Reducing Measles Mortality, Reducing Child Mortality. *Lancet* 368:1050–1053.

Hopkins, Donald R. 1983. *The Greatest Killer: Smallpox in History*. Chicago: University of Chicago Press.

Hopkins, Donald R., Ernesto Ruiz-Tiben, Philip Downs, P. Craig Withers, and Sharon Roy. 2007. Dracunculiasis Eradication: Neglected No Longer. *American Journal of Tropical Medicine and Hygiene* 79:474–479.

Hopkins, Jack W. 1989. *The Eradication of Smallpox*. Boulder, Colo.: Westview Press.

Horstmann, Dorothy M. 1984. Preface. *Reviews of Infectious Diseases* 6:S301.

Hull, H. F., Nicholas Ward, Barbara P. Hull, Julie B. Milstein, and Ciro de Quadros. 1994. Paralytic Poliomyelitis: Seasoned Strategies, Disappearing Disease. *Lancet* 343:1331–1337.

Hyder, Adnan A., and Richard H. Morrow. 2000. Applying Burden of Disease Methods in Developing Countries: A Case Study from Pakistan. *American Journal of Public Health* 90:1235–1240.

Imperato, Pascal James. 2001. Global Health. *Journal of Community Health* 26:77.

Islam, Nasir. 2004. Sifarish, Sycophants, Power and Collectivism: Administrative Culture in Pakistan. *International Review of Administrative Sciences* 70:311–330.

Jegede, Ayodele Samuel. 2007. What Led to the Nigerian Boycott of the Polio Vaccination Campaign? *Public Library of Science Medicine* 4:e73.

Jenney, E. R., and O. G. Simmons. 1954. Human Relations and Technical Assistance in Public Health. *Scientific Monthly* 78:365–371.

Jian, Zhang, Yu Jing-jin, Zhang Rong-zhen, Zhang Xing-lu, Zhou Jun, et al. 1998. Costs of Polio Immunization Days in China: Implications for Mass Immunization Campaign Strategies. *International Journal of Health Planning and Management* 13:5–25.

John, J. 1984. Poliomyelitis in India: Prospects and Problems of Control. *Reviews of Infectious Diseases* 6:S438–S441.

Jordan, William S. 1984. Prospects for Worldwide Control of Paralytic Poliomyelitis: A Discussion. *Reviews of Infectious Diseases* 6:S594-S595.

Justice, Judith. 1986. *Policies, Plans, and People*. Berkeley: University of California Press.

Ke-an, Wang, Zhang Li-bi, Mac W. Otten, Zhang Xing-lu, Yasuo Chiba, et al. 1997. Status of the Eradication of Indigenous Wild Poliomyelitis in the People's Republic of China. *Journal of Infectious Diseases* 175:S105–112.

Keefer, Philip E., Ambar Narayan, and Tara Vishwanath. 2003. The Political Economy of Decentralization in Pakistan. Washington, D.C.: Development Research Group, World Bank. *sticerd.lse.ac.uk/dps/decentralisation/Pakistan.pdf.*

Keller, Evelyn Fox. 1985. *Reflections on Gender and Science*. New Haven: Yale University Press.

Keller, Evelyn Fox, and Helen Longino, eds. 1996. *Feminism and Science*. Oxford: Oxford University Press.

Kelly-Hope, Louise, Hilary Ranson, and Janet Hemingway. 2008. Lessons from the Past: Managing Insecticide Resistance in Malaria Control and Eradication Programs. *Lancet Infectious Diseases* 8:387–89.

Kew, Olen, Victoria Morris-Glasgow, Mauricio Landaverde, Cara Burns, Jing Shaw, et al. 2002. Outbreak of Poliomyelitis in Hispaniola Associated with Circulating Type 1 Vaccine-Derived Poliovirus. *Science* 296:356–359.

Khan, M. M., and J. Ehreth. 2003. Costs and Benefits of Polio Eradication: A Long-Run Global Perspective. *Vaccine* 21:702–5.

Khan, Muhammad Nasir. 2004. Presidential Address. Second Plenary Meeting, Fifty-seventh World Health Assembly. Geneva: WHO.

*Lancet*. 2007. Is Malaria Eradication Possible? *Lancet* 370:1459.

Lee, J. W., Bjorn Melgaard, H. F. Hull, D. Barakamfitiye, and J. M. Okwo-Bele. 1998. On the Other Hand: Ethical Dilemmas in Polio Eradication. *American Journal of Public Health* 88:130–131.

Levin, Ann, Sujata Ram, and Miloud Kaddar. 2002. The Impact of the Global Polio Eradication Initiative on the Financing of Routine Immunization: Case Studies in Bangladesh, Côte d'Ivoire, and Morocco. *Bulletin of the World Health Organization* 80:822–828.

Lewis, David. 2004. On the Difficulty of Studying "Civil Society": Reflections on NGOs, State and Democracy in Bangladesh. *Contributions to Indian Sociology* 38:299–322.

Li, Tania. 2007. *The Will to Improve*. Durham, N.C.: Duke University Press.

Little, Peter, and Michael Painter. 1995. Discourse, Politics, and the Development Process: Reflections on Escobar's "Anthropology and the Development Encounter." *American Ethnologist* 22:602–616.

Lockwood, Diana, and Sujai Suneetha. 2005. Leprosy: Too Complex a Disease for a Simple Elimination Paradigm. *Bulletin of the World Health Organization* 83.

Loevinsohn, Benjamin, Bruce Aylward, Robert Steinglass, Ellyn Ogden, Tracey Goodman, and B. Melgaard. 2002. Impact of Targeted Programs on Health Systems: A Case Study of the Polio Eradication Initiative. *American Journal of Public Health* 92:19–23.

Losos, J. 1999. Report of the Workgroup on Viral Diseases. *Morbidity and Mortality Weekly Report* 48:126–137.

Lowther, S. A., T. Mir, K. Bile, R. Hafiz, and A. W. Mounts. 2002. Characteristics of Districts and District Health Officials in Pakistan as Potential Predictors of Persistent Transmission of Wild Poliovirus, 2000–2001. Author files.

Lowy, Ilana. 1997. Epidemiology, Immunology, and Yellow Fever: The Rockefeller Foundation in Brazil, 1923–1939. *Journal of the History of Biology* 30:397–417.

Macdonald, George. 1965. Eradication of Malaria. *Public Health Reports* 80:870–879.

Mahler, Halfdan. 1988. Provisional Verbatim Record of the Seventh Plenary Meeting. Forty-First World Health Assembly. Geneva.

Malinowski, Bronislaw. 1922. *Argonauts of the Western Pacific*. New York: E. P. Dutton.

Maqbool, Shahina. 2005. Pakistan to Precision Target the Most Stubborn Strain of Poliovirus. *News* (Rawalpindi/Islamabad) 2 September.

Marcus, George. 1995. Ethnography in/of the World System: The Emergence of Multi-Sited Ethnography. *Annual Review of Anthropology* 24:95–117.

Markowitz, L. 2001. Finding the Field: Notes on the Ethnography of NGOs. *Human Organization* 39:183–203.

Mauss, Marcel. 1967. *The Gift*. New York: W. W. Norton.

Mayes, Bronston T., and Robert W. Allen. 1977. Toward a Definition of Organizational Politics. *Academy of Management Review* 2:672–678.

McBean, A. M., M. L. Thoms, and P. Albrecht. 1988. Serologic Response to Oral Polio Vaccine and Enhanced-Potency Inactivated Polio Vaccines. *American Journal of Epidemiology* 128:615–628.

McFarland, Deborah A. 1995. The Economics of Global Disease Eradication. In *World Health Day: Target 2000: A World without Polio*: World Health Organization. *whqlibdoc.who.int/hq/1995/WHD_95.1-8.pdf.*

McNeil, Donald G. 2008. Eradicate Malaria? Doubters Fuel Debate. *New York Times*, March 4.

———. 2009. Global Fund Is Billions Short. *New York Times* 2 February.

Measles Initiative. 2009. Key Statistics. *measlesinitiative.org/docs/mi-key-statistics.pdf.*

Meissner, H. Cody, Peter M. Strebel, and W. A. Orenstein. 2004. Measles Vaccines and the Potential for Worldwide Eradication of Measles. *Pediatrics* 114:1065–1069.

Mendis, Kamini, Aafje Rietvelt, Marian Warsame, Andrea Bosman, Brian Greenwood, and Walther Wernsdorfer. 2009. From Malaria Control to Eradication: The WHO Perspective. *Tropical Medicine and International Health* 14:1–7.

Menon, R., and K. Bhasin. 1998. *Borders and Boundaries: Women in India's Partition.* New Brunswick, N.J.: Rutgers University Press.

Miller, Mark, Scott Barrett, and D. A. Henderson. 2006. Control and Eradication. In *Disease Control Priorities in Developing Countries*, 2nd ed., ed. Jamison et al., 1163–1176. New York: Oxford University Press.

Mitchell, Timothy. 1990. Everyday Metaphors of Power. *Theory and Society* 19:545–577.

Morgan, Lynn. 1989. "Political Will" and Community Participation in Costa Rican Primary Health Care. *Medical Anthropology Quarterly* 3:232–245.

Mosse, David. 2005. *Cultivating Development.* London: Pluto Books.

Muraskin, William. 1998. *The Politics of International Health: The Children's Vaccine Initiative and the Struggle to Develop Vaccines for the Third World.* Albany: State University of New York Press.

Muscat, Mark, Henrik Bang, Jan Wohlfahrt, Steffen Glismann, and Kare Melbak. 2009. Measles in Europe: An Epidemiological Assessment. *Lancet* 373:383–389.

Nakano, Takashi, Zheng-Rong Ding, Zhi-Song Liang, Tsuyoshi Matsuba, and Wen Xu. 1997. Transient Population Bypassed by Polio Vaccination Programmes in Yunnan Province, China. *The Lancet* 350:1004.

Needham, Cynthia, and Richard Canning. 2003. *Global Disease Eradication: The Race for the Last Child.* Washington, D.C.: ASM Press.

Nguyen, Vinh-Kim, and Karine Peschard. 2003. Anthropology, Inequality, and Disease: A Review. *Annual Review of Anthropology* 32:447–74.

Nichter, Mark. 1996. The Primary Health Center as a Social System: Primary Health Care, Social Status, and the Issue of Team-work in South Asia. In *Anthropology and International Health: Asian Case Studies*, ed. M. Nichter, 367–391. Amsterdam: Gordon and Breach.

Okie, Susan. 2008. A New Attack on Malaria. *New England Journal of Medicine* 358:2425.

Orenstein, W. A., Peter M. Strebel, Mark Papania, R. W. Sutter, William J. Bellini, and S. L. Cochi. 2000. Measles Eradication: Is It in Our Future? *American Journal of Public Health* 90:1521–1525.

Oshinsky, David M. 2005. *Polio: An American Story*. New York: Oxford University Press.

Packard, Randall. 1997. Malaria Dreams: Postwar Visions of Health and Development in the Third World. *Medical Anthropology* 17:279–296.

Packard, Randall, and Peter J. Brown. 1997. Rethinking Health, Development, and Malaria: Historicizing a Cultural Model in International Health. *Medical Anthropology* 17:181–194.

Pallansch, Mark A., and Hardeep S. Sandhu. 2006. The Eradication of Polio— Progress and Challenges. *New England Journal of Medicine* 55:2508–2511.

Pan American Health Organization. 1994. Measles Elimination by the Year 2000! *EPI Newsletter* 16:1–2.

———. 1995. The Impact of the Expanded Program on Immunization and the Polio Eradication Initiative on Health Systems in the Americas: Final Report of the "Taylor Commission." Washington, D.C.: PAHO.

———. 2009. Measles Elimination, the Americas, 2001–2009. *Measles/Rubella Weekly Bulletin* 15(22): 1. *new.paho.org/hq/index.php?option=com_docman &Itemid=673*.

Paul, Benjamin. 1955. *Health, Culture, and Community*. New York: Russell Sage.

Pfeiffer, James. 2004. International NGOs in the Mozambique Health Sector: The "Velvet Glove" of Privatization. In *Unhealthy Health Policy*, ed. A. Castro, M. Singer. Walnut Creek, Calif.: AltaMira Press.

Pigman, Herbert A. 2005. *Conquering Polio: A Brief History of PolioPlus, Rotary's Role in a Global Program to Eradicate the World's Greatest Crippling Disease*. Evanston, Ill.: Rotary International.

Platts, John T. 2004. *A Dictionary of Urdu, Classical Hindi, and English*. New Delhi: Munshiram Manoharlal.

Post, Thierry, Martijn van den Assem, Guido Baltussen, and Richard H. Thaler. 2007. Deal or No Deal? Decision Making under Risk in a Large-Payoff Game Show. *ssrn.com/abstract=636508*.

Rafei, Uton Muchtar. 1995. Message from Dr. Uton Muchtar Rafei, Regional Director, WHO South-East Asia Region, on the Occasion of World Health Day 1995. Geneva: WHO. *whqlibdoc.who.int/hq/1995/WHD_95.1-8.pdf*.

Ravishankar, Nirmala, Paul Gubbins, Rebecca Cooley, Katherine Leach-Kemon, Catherine Michaud, et al. 2009. Financing of Global Health: Tracking Development Assistance for Health from 1990 to 2007. *Lancet* 373:2113–2124.

Renne, Elisha. 2006. Perspectives on Polio and Immunization in Northern Nigeria. *Social Science and Medicine* 63:1857–1869.

Risi, Joao Baptista, Jr. 1997. Poliomyelitis in Brazil. In *Polio*, ed. T. M. Daniel, F. C. Robbins, 159–180. Rochester, N.Y.: Rochester University Press.

Robbins, Frederick C. 1984. Summary and Recommendations. *Reviews of Infectious Diseases* 6:S596–S600.

Roberts, Leslie. 2006. Polio Eradication: Is It Time to Give Up? *Science* 312:832–835.

———. 2007. Vaccine-Related Polio Outbreak in Nigeria Raises Concerns. *Science* 317:1842.

Roberts, Leslie, and Martin Enserink. 2007. Did They Really Say . . . Eradication? *Science* 318:1544–1545.

Rogers, John D. 1991. Cultural and Social Resistance: Gambling in Colonial Sri Lanka. In *Contesting Power*, ed. D. Haynes, G. Prakash, 175–212. Berkeley: University of California Press.

Rotary Foundation. 1985. PolioPlus Programme: Criteria for Funding of Polio Immunization Programmes. *Assignment Children* 69–72:187–92.

Russell, Paul F. 1955. *Man's Mastery of Malaria*. London: Oxford University Press.

Sabin, Albert B. 1984. Strategies for Elimination of Poliomyelitis in Different Parts of the World with Use of Oral Poliovirus Vaccine. *Reviews of Infectious Diseases* 6:S391–S396.

Sachs, Jeffrey D. 2005. *The End of Poverty*. New York: Penguin Press.

Sangrujee, N., V. M. Caceres, and S. L. Cochi. 2004. Cost Analysis of Post-Polio Certification Immunization Policies. *Bulletin of the World Health Organization* 82:9–15.

Scott, James C. 1969. The Analysis of Corruption in Developing Nations. *Comparative Studies in Society and History* 11:315–341.

———. 1972. Patron-Client Politics and Political Change in Southeast Asia. *American Political Science Review* 66:91–113.

———. 1985. *Weapons of the Weak*. New Haven: Yale University Press.

———. 1990. *Domination and the Arts of Resistance*. New Haven: Yale University Press.

Seytre, Bernard, and Mary Shaffer. 2005. *The Death of a Disease: A History of the Eradication of Poliomyelitis*. New Brunswick, N.J.: Rutgers University Press.

Sharma, Aradhana. 2006. Crossbreeding Institutions, Breeding Struggle: Women's Empowerment, Neoliberal Governmentality, and State (Re)Formation in India. *Cultural Anthropology* 21:60–95.

Sharma, Aradhana, and Akhil Gupta. 2006. Introduction: Rethinking Theories of the State in an Age of Globalization. In *The Anthropology of the State*, ed. A. Sharma, A. Gupta, 1–42. Malden, Mass.: Blackwell.

Singer, Merrill. 1998. Beyond the Ivory Tower: Critical Praxis in Medical Anthropology. In *Understanding and Applying Medical Anthropology*, ed. P. J. Brown, 225–239. Mountain View, Calif.: Mayfield Publishing.

Singer, Merrill, Freddie Valentin, Hans Baer, and Zhongke Jia. 1992. Why Does Juan Garcia Have a Drinking Problem? The Perspective of Critical Medical Anthropology. *Medical Anthropology* 14:77–108.

Sivaramakrishnan, K. 2005. Some Intellectual Geneaologies for the Concept of Everyday Resistance. *American Anthropologist* 107:346–355.

Smallman-Raynor, M. R., A. D. Cliff, B. Trevelyan, C. Nettleton, and S. Sneddon. 2006. *Poliomyelitis: Emergence to Eradication*. Oxford: Oxford University Press.

Smith, Daniel Jordan. 2001. Kinship and Corruption in Contemporary Nigeria. *Ethnos* 66:344–364.

———. 2003. Patronage, Per Diems and the "Workshop Mentality": The Practice of Family Planning Programs in Southeastern Nigeria. *World Development* 31:703–715.

———. 2007. *A Culture of Corruption*. Princeton: Princeton University Press.

Soper, Fred L. 1963. Elimination of Urban Yellow Fever. *American Journal of Public Health* 53:7–16.

———. 1965. Rehabilitation of the Eradication Concept in Prevention of Communicable Diseases. *Public Health Reports* 80:855–869.

Staw, Barry M. 1976. Knee-Deep in the Big Muddy: A Study of Escalating Commitment to a Chosen Course of Action. *Organizational Behavior and Human Performance* 16:27–44.

———. 1981. The Escalation of Commitment to a Course of Action. *Academy of Management Review* 6:577–587.

Sutter, R. W., and S. L. Cochi. 1997. Comment: Ethical Dilemmas in Worldwide Polio Eradication Programs. *American Journal of Public Health* 87:913–916.

Tayeh, Ahmed, and Sandy Cairncross. 2007. Editorial: Dracunculiasis Eradication by 2009: Will Endemic Countries Meet the Target? *Tropical Medicine and International Health* 12:1403–1408.

Taylor, Carl E., Felicity Cutts, and Mary E. Taylor. 1997. Ethical Dilemmas in Current Planning for Polio Eradication. *American Journal of Public Health* 87:922–925.

Technical Advisory Group on Polio Eradication in Pakistan and Afghanistan. 2001. Draft Conclusions and Recommendations, November 27–29, Cairo, Egypt. *emro.who.int/polio/meetings/TAGpak/Second%20TAG%20Pak.pdf.*

Technical Advisory Groups on Polio Eradication in Afghanistan and in Pakistan. 2007. Conclusions and Recommendations, April 17–18, Islamabad. *polioeradication.org/content/meetings/FinalReportJointAFGPAKTAGApril2007.pdf.*

Tendler, Judith. 1975. *Inside Foreign Aid.* Baltimore, Md.: Johns Hopkins University Press.

Thaler, Richard H., and Eric J. Johnson. 1990. Gambling with the House Money and Trying to Break Even: The Effects of Prior Outcomes on Risky Choice. *Managment Science* 36:643–660.

Thigpen, Scott, dir. 2004. *The Last Child: The Global Race to End Polio.* USA: Red Sky Productions.

Thompson, Kimberly M., and Radboud J. Duintjer Tebbens. 2007. Eradication versus Control for Poliomyelitis: An Economic Analysis. *Lancet* 369:1363–1371.

Tiger, Lionel. 1979. *Optimism: The Biology of Hope.* New York: Kodansha International.

Transparency International. 2002. Corruption in South Asia. Transparency International. *unpan1.un.org/intradoc/groups/public/documents/APCITY/UNPAN019883.pdf.*

———. 2008. *Corruption Perceptions Index 2007. transparency.org/policy_research/surveys_indices/cpi/2007.*

Tucker, Jonathan B. 2001. *Scourge: The Once and Future Threat of Smallpox.* New York: Grove Press.

UNICEF. 1996. Sustainability of Achievements: Lessons Learned from Universal Child Immunization. New York: UNICEF.

———. 2000. Reaching the Last Child with Polio Vaccine. Press release. *unicef.org/newsline/00prpolio.htm.*

United Nations. 2007. The Millennium Development Goals Report 2007. New York: United Nations. *un.org/millenniumgoals/pdf/mdg2007.pdf.*

U.S. Congress. 1999. Global Eradication of Polio and Measles. Special Hearing 105-883, Committee on Appropriations Subcommittee, 105th Cong., 2d Sess. Washington, D.C.: U.S. Government Printing Office.

Verkaaik, Oskar. 2001. The Captive State: Corruption, Intelligence Agencies, and Ethnicity in Pakistan. In *States of Imagination: Ethnographic Explorations of the Postcolonial State*, ed. T. B. Hansen, F. Stepputat, 345–364. Durham, N.C.: Duke University Press.

Walker, Stephen L., and Roderick J. Hay. 2001. Yaws—A Review of the Last 50 Years. *International Journal of Dermatology* 39:258–260.

Ward, Nicholas, and H. F. Hull. 1995. Towards TARGET 2000: A Polio Eradication Progress Report. In *Target 2000: A World without Polio: World Health Day*. Geneva: WHO. *whqlibdoc.who.int/hq/1995/WHD_95.1-8.pdf.*

Ward, Nicholas, Julie B. Milstein, H. F. Hull, Barbara P. Hull, and R. J. Kim-Farley. 1993. The WHO-EPI Initiative for the Global Eradication of Poliomyelitis. *Biologicals* 21:327–333.

Weber, Max. 1978. *Economy and Society*. Berkeley: University of California Press.

Weingrod, Alex. 1968. Patrons, Patronage, and Political Parties. *Comparative Studies in Society and History* 10:377–400.

Werner, Cynthia. 2000. Gifts, Bribes, and Development in Post-Soviet Kazakhstan. *Human Organization* 59:11–22.

Wolf, Eric. 1966. Kinship, Friendship, and Patron-Client Relations. In *The Social Anthropology of Complex Societies*, ed. M. Banton, 1–22. London: Tavistock Publications.

———. 1982. *Europe and the People without History*. Berkeley: University of California Press.

———. 1990. Distinguished Lecture: Facing Power—Old Insights, New Questions. *American Anthropologist* 92:586–596.

World Health Assembly. 1988. Global Eradication of Poliomyelitis by the Year 2000. *Forty-First World Health Assembly*. Geneva, 2–13 May.

World Health Organization. 1978. Declaration of Alma-Ata. *International Conference on Primary Health Care*. Alma-Ata, USSR. *who.int/hpr/NPH/docs/ declaration_almaata.pdf.*

———. 1988. Global Poliomyelitis Eradication by the Year 2000: Plan of Action. Geneva: WHO.

———. 1990. Eradication of Poliomyelitis: Report of the Third Consultation. Geneva: WHO.

———. 1992. Report of the Technical Consultative Group Meeting with Special Focus on the Global Eradication of Poliomyelitis. Geneva: WHO.

———. 1995a. A World without Polio: Target 2000. Geneva: WHO. *whqlibdoc.who.int/hq/1995/WHD_95.1-8.pdf.*

———. 1995b. In Point of Fact. In *Target 2000: A World without Polio: World Health Day 1995*, 31–34. Geneva: WHO. *whqlibdoc.who.int/hq/1995/ WHD_95.1-8.pdf.*

———. 1996. Global Poliomyelitis Eradication by the Year 2000. Geneva: WHO.

———. 1997. Polio: The Beginning of the End. Geneva: WHO.

———. 1998a. Global Eradication of Poliomyelitis: Report of the Third Meeting of the Global Commission for the Certification of the Eradication of Polio, Geneva, 9 July 1998. Geneva: WHO.

———. 1998b. Report of the Second Meeting of the Global Commission for the Certification of the Eradication of Poliomyelitis. Geneva: WHO.

————. 2001a. Global Polio Eradication Initiative Estimated External Financial Resource Requirements for 2002–2005. Geneva: WHO. *whqlibdoc.who.int/hq/2001/WHO_POLIO_01.05.pdf.*

————. 2001b. Global Polio Eradication Progress 2000. Geneva: WHO.

————. 2002. Global Polio Eradication Initiative Progress 2001. Geneva: WHO.

————. 2003. Global Polio Eradication Initiative Strategic Plan 2004–2008. Geneva: WHO. *www.polioeradication.org/content/publications/004stratplan.pdf.*

————. 2004. Global Polio Eradication Initiative Progress 2003. Geneva: WHO.

————. 2005a. Global Polio Eradication Initiative 2004 Annual Report, Geneva: WHO.

————. 2005b. Global Polio Eradication Initiative Financial Resource Requirements 2005 to 2008. Geneva: WHO.

————. 2005c. Report of an Informal Technical Consultation on Polio Eradication in Pakistan. Islamabad: WHO. *polioeradication.org/content/general/PAK_May_05%20Inf_tech_consult_report.pdf.*

————. 2006a. Conclusions and Recommendations of the Advisory Committee on Poliomyelitis Eradication, Geneva, 11–12 October 2006, Part II. *Weekly Epidemiological Record* 81:465–468.

————. 2006b. Global Polio Eradication Initiative Financial Resource Requirements 2006–2008 as of September 2006. Geneva: World Health Organization.

————. 2006c. Global Polio Eradication Now Hinges on Four Countries. *Polio News*:1.

————. 2006d. Global Polio Eradication Now Hinges on Four Countries: Polio-Free Countries Seek to Protect Themselves. News Release WHO/56. Geneva: WHO. *whqlibdoc.who.int/press_release/2006/PR_56.pdf.*

————. 2006e. Pakistan Mortality Country Fact Sheet 2006.Cairo: WHO Eastern Mediterranean Region (EMRO). *who.int/whosis/mort/profiles/mort_emro_pak_pakistan.pdf.*

————. 2006f. Progress Report on Polio Eradication, Eastern Mediterranean Region. Cairo: WHO.

————. 2006g. Progress towards Polio Eradication in Afghanistan and Pakistan, January 2005 to May 2006. *Weekly Epidemiological Record* 81:241–248.

————. 2006h. Provisional Summary Record of the Second Meeting. *Fifty-Ninth World Health Assembly.* Geneva: WHO.

————. 2007a. Global Polio Eradication Initiative Annual Report 2006. Geneva: WHO. *polioeradication.org/content/publications/AnnualReport2006_ENG.pdf.*

————. 2007b. World Health Statistics 2007. Geneva: WHO.

————. 2008a. Dracunculiasis Eradication: Global Surveillance Summary, 2007. *Weekly Epidemiological Record* 18:159–167.

————. 2008b. Global Polio Eradication Initiative Financial Resource Requirements 2008–2012 as of January 2008. Geneva: WHO.

————. 2008c. World Health Statistics 2008. Geneva: WHO. *who.int/whosis/whostat/2008/en/index.html.*

————. 2009. Monthly Report on Dracunculiasis Cases, January–April 2009. *Weekly Epidemiological Record* 84:212.

World Health Organization, Rotary International, CDC, and UNICEF. 2007. Polio
    Eradication: Review of the Strategies and Feasibility. Presentation at the Urgent
    Stakeholders' Meeting, Geneva, February 2007. *polioeradication.org/content/
    meetings/Strategies&feasibility.pdf.*
Yang, Baoping, Jian Zhang, Mac W. Otten, Kazuo Kusumoto, Tao Jiang, et al.
    1995. Eradication of Poliomyelitis: Progress in the People's Republic of China.
    *Pediatric Infectious Disease Journal* 14:308–314.
Zhang, Jian, Li-bi Zhang, Mac W. Otten, Jiang Tae, Zhang Xing-lu, et al. 1997.
    Surveillance for Polio Eradication in the People's Republic of China. *The Journal
    of Infectious Diseases* 175:S122–34.

# Index

*Page numbers in bold refer to photo captions.*

CPSIA information can be obtained
at www.ICGtesting.com
Printed in the USA
LVHW111821050120
642561LV00001B/84/P